Advances in Stereotactic and Functional Neurosurgery 9

Proceedings of the 9th Meeting of the European Society for Stereotactic and Functional Neurosurgery, Malaga 1990

Edited by
E. R. Hitchcock, G. Broggi, J. Burzaco, J. Martin-Rodriguez, B. A. Meyerson, Sz. Tóth

Acta Neurochirurgica Supplementum 52

Springer-Verlag Wien New York

Professor Edward R. Hitchcock
Department of Neurosurgery, University of Birmingham, U.K.

Prof. Dr. Giovanni Broggi
Istituto Neurologico "C. Besta", Milano, Italy

Dr. Juan Burzaco
Servicio de Neurocirugía, Fundación Iménez Díaz, Madrid, Spain

Dr. J. Martin-Rodriguez
Fundacion "Sixto Obrador", Dept. de Neurocirurgia, Madrid, Spain

Dr. Björn A. Meyerson
Department of Neurosurgery, Karolinska Sjukhuset, Stockholm, Sweden

Dr. Szabolcs Tóth
Department of Neurosurgery, Medical University of Debrecen, Debrecen, Hungary

With 67 Figures

Typesetting: Thomson Press, New Delhi, India
Printed in Germany by K. Triltsch, Würzburg

Printed on acid-free paper

ISSN 0065-1419 (Acta Neurochirurgica/Suppl.)
ISSN 0720-7972 (Advances in Stereotactic and Functional Neurosurgery)
ISBN 3-211-82283-6 Springer-Verlag Wien-New York
ISBN 0-387-82283-6 Springer-Verlag New York-Wien

Contents

Listed in Current Contents

Technical Contributions

Brain Tumours, Stereotactical and Radiosurgical Management

Movement Disorder

Thalamic and Dorsal Column Stimulation

Pain

Biological Research in Psychiatry

Epilepsy

“In Situ” Drugs Administration

Acta Neurochirurgica, Suppl. 52, 3–4 (1991)

Toxicology and Kinetics of Long-Term Intraventricular Infusion of Phenytoin and Valproic Acid in Pigs: Experimental Study

R. Martínez, J. Vaquero, L.V. De La Morena[1], F. Tendillo[2], and P. Aragonés

Departments of Neurosurgery, [1]Pharmacology, and [2]Experimental Surgery, Puerta de Hierro Clinic, Autonomous University of Madrid, Madrid, Spain

Summary

The effect of continuous intraventricular infusion of phenytoin and valproic acid into the brain of pigs was studied through quantitative measurement of animal behavior, pathological study of animal's brain and measurement of the levels of these drugs in the blood and C.S.F. Two groups of five animals each were treated with increasingly doses of the drugs until the apparition of toxic effects and the dead of animals. Normal behavior was observed with doses up to 3 mg/day of phenytoin and 1.5 mg/day of valproic acid. Toxic effects consisted on severe unsteadiness and muscular rigidity. Pathological study of the brains revealed that there were no damage attributable to the intraventricular infusion of the drugs. The present study suggests that intrathecal or intraventricular infusion of phenytoin and valproic acid could be well tolerated by humans and it leads us to consider subsequent clinical studies in epileptic patients.

Keywords: Phenytoin; valproic acid; intraventricular infusion; epilepsy.

Introduction

Intraventricular infusion of antiepileptic drugs might be a useful treatment in selected epileptic patients. The limited number of previous reports have shown that concentrations in the cerebrospinal fluid (CSF) of antiepileptic drugs reach 10% of serum concentrations at most[2,3] and that intrathecal delivery of antiepileptic drugs controls experimental seizures in animal models[1].

The present study was designed to determine the behavioral and pathological changes induced by the continuous intraventricular infusion of phenytoin and valproic acid in pigs.

Materials and Methods

Adult pigs of 25 kg were selected for this study because the ventricular ependyma, cerebral cortex and cerebellar tissue in this animal have features common with the human brain. Intraventricular implantation of a catheter connected to a subcutaneously implanted infusion pump* was performed on ten pigs divided in two groups of five animals each.

Each group of animals was treated with increasing doses of phenytoin and valproic acid respectively. The doses were reviewed weekly according to the animal behavior and to the levels of the drugs in the blood and CSF of the animals. The doses were increased until the appearence of toxic effects and death of the animals.

Quantitative measurement of the animals' behavior was done by observation of alimentary rhythms, gait and irritability to different stimuli (light and pain). When these functions were unchanged after the operation, they were considered as "normal". The appearence of gait unsteadiness changes of alimentary of behavior and slowing of responses to light and pain were interpreted as toxic effects.

The stability of the drug solutions was reviewed regularly and maintained throughout the experiment.

When the animals died, the brains were removed rapidly, cut into 6 mm coronal slices and fixed in formalin. The sections were then prepared for light microscopy by staining with hematoxylin and eosin.

Results

The animals showed normal behavior with mean doses up to 3 mg/day of phenytoin and 1.5 mg/day of valproic acid (Fig. 1). Toxic effects consisted of muscle rigidity, unsteadiness and progressive stupor until death.

Histology of the brains showed no changes as compared to brains of non-treated animals, both with regard to cerebellum, cerebral cortex and ependymal epithelium.

* "Infusaid-500" pump. Shiley Infusaid Inc., Mass., USA.

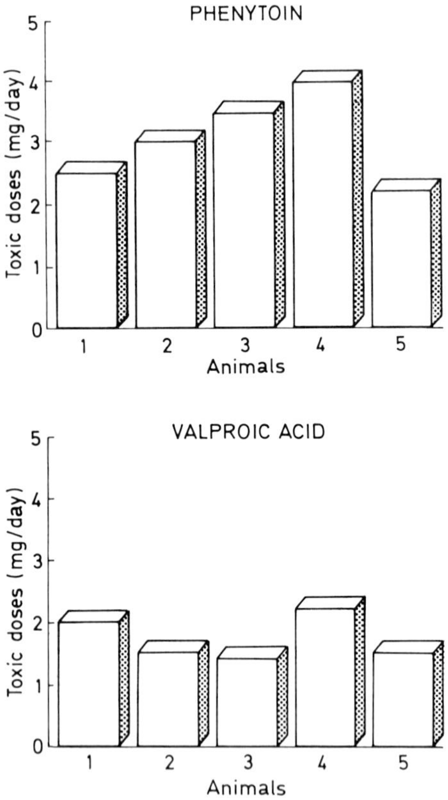

Fig. 1. Histograms showing the toxic doses in each animal

Discussion

It has been reported that intrathecal administration of antiepileptic drugs may effectively control seizures in an epileptic animal model[1]. In most patients treated with oral medication of antiepileptic drugs the concentration in CSF is about 10% of the serum levels[2,3].

In selected cases, such as patients with seizures resistant to oral medication or with important systemic side effects related to antiepileptic drugs, continuous intraventricular or intrathecal infusion of these drugs could be an alternative treatment.

The present study shows that intraventricular infusion of phenytoin and valproic acid does not seem to be cause of damage to the nervous system as shown by the lack of obvious histological changes. Toxic doses have been defined in each individual animal. These results lead us to consider a clinical study with intrathecal administration of antiepileptic drugs.

References

1. Gonzalez-Dader JM, Guerrero M, Esteban J (1989) Intrathecal infusion of antiepileptic drugs. An experimental study. Acta Neurochir (Wien) 98: 100
2. Vadja FJE, Williams FM, Davidson S, Breckenridge A (1974) Human brain, cerebrospinal fluid and plasma concentration of diphenylhydantoin and phenobarbital. Clin Pharmacol Ther 15: 597–603
3. Vadja FJE, Donnan GA, Phillips J, Blandin PF (1981) Human brain, plasma and cerebrospinal fluid concentrations of sodium valproate after 72 hours of therapy. Neurology 31: 486–487.

Correspondence: Dr. R. Martínez, Servicio de Neurocirugía, Clínica Puerta de Hierro, C/San Martín de Porres 4, E-28035 Madrid, Spain.

Acta Neurochirurgica, Suppl. 52, 5–6 (1991)

Antinociceptive Activity of Intracerebroventricular Lysine Acetylsalicylate: An Experimental Study

M. Meglio, B. Cioni, A. Moles, A. Puca, and **M. Visocchi**

Istituto di Neurochirurgia, Università Cattolica, Roma, Italy

Summary

We investigated the antinociceptive activity of Lysine Acetylsalicylate (LAS) after intracerebroventricular (icv) injection in experimental animals. The effect on tonic pain was studied by means of the Formalin test on 140 male Swiss mice. In a first group of animals icv LAS was injected at different doses (0.25–0.5–1 mg in saline solution 5 μl). A second group received icv morphine 1 μg in 5μl saline, and finally a third control group received icv 5 μl saline. The effect of the compounds on the Formalin test was evaluated under blind conditions.

Icv LAS had no effect on the nociceptive behaviour at doses of 0.25 and 0.5 mg, while a reduction of the licking time was evident after the injection of 1 mg of the drug. The time course and the degree of the analgesic effect of icv LAS was investigated and compared to the effect of icv morphine.

Keywords: Experimental pain; lysine Acetylsalicylate; intracerebroventricular administration.

Introduction

Remarkable and long lasting analgesia after intrathecal injection of Lysine Acetylsalicylate (LAS) in man was reported by Devoghel[1] and by Pellerin *et al.*[3]. Encouraged by such reports, we decided to evaluate this drug as an alternative to morphine. Unfortunately, we could not reproduce good results in our first six patients and therefore decided to investigate in experimental animals the antinociceptive activity of LAS after intracerebroventricular (icv) injection.

Material and Methods

Animals and Drugs

140 male Swiss mice (25–35 gr; housed 5 per cage with 12 hr light cycle; food and water ad libitum) were used. Under light ether anesthesia, the mice received icv injection (transcutaneous puncture 1–2 mm behind the bregma on the midline, 4 mm depth) of different drugs in an equal volume of 5 μl vehicle.

A first group of animals was injected with icv LAS at different concentrations (LAS 0.25, 0.5 and 1 mg in saline solution 5 μl). A second group received icv morphine chloride 1 μg in saline 5 μl; and finally a third control group received icv saline solution 5 μl. The dosage of icv LAS and morphine was calculated on the basis of the ratio mouse and man brain weight: icv LAS 1 mg in mouse is approximate equal to LAS 1–1.3 g in man, and icv morphine 1 μg in mouse equals morphine 1–1.3 mg in man. Each mouse was used on one occasion only.

Evaluation of Antinociceptive Activity

We used the Formalin test[2] as a model of tonic pain. The noxious stimulus was the injection of 20 μl of 5% Formalin under the skin of the dorsal surface of the right hindpaw, using a minimum of restraint. The mouse was then placed into the observation chamber (Plexiglas cage 30 cm × 20 cm × 13 cm). The amount of time in seconds the animal spent licking the injected paw was recorded during a time window +20 min to +40 min starting from the Formalin injection, and was regarded as the nociceptive response.

Formalin was injected at different times after icv administration of the test drugs (0′–60′–120′–180′).

The effect of the compounds on the Formalin test was evaluated under blind conditions.

Analysis of Data

Experimental groups each consisted of 10–21 animals.

The results were expressed as mean +/− standard error of the mean. Data were analysed by analysis o variance (ANOVA) followed by single comparisons of means (2-tailed tests).

Results

The animals of the control group (icv saline 5 μl) spent 118.4 +/− 19.32 seconds licking their hindpaw.

The animals of the morphine group spent 23.4 +/− 8.25 sec. In this group, the licking time was thus significantly lower than in the control group.

Icv LAS had no effect on the nociceptive behaviour at doses of 0.25 and 0.5 mg (licking time 115.4 +/−

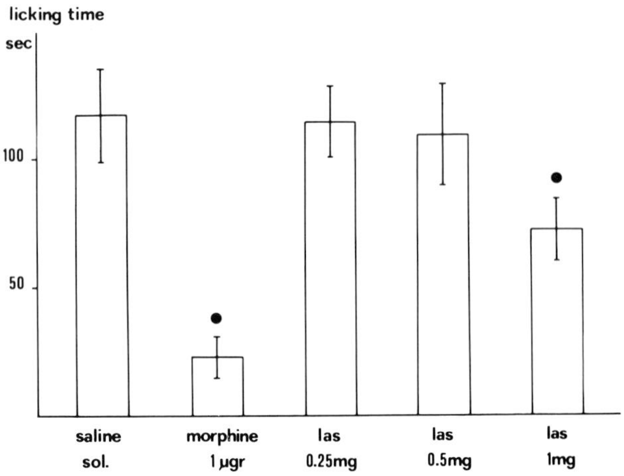

Fig. 1. The antinociceptive activity of icv LAS at different doses and of morphine compared to matched saline control group. The nociceptive response (licking time) is expressed as mean and standard error of mean. The black spots indicate significantly lower paw licking ($p = 0.0002$ for morphine and $p = 0.05$ for LAS)

14.74 and 110.4 +/− 20.09 sec, respectively). A significant reduction of the licking time was evident after the injection of 1 mg of the drug (73.4 +/− 12.46 sec).

The analgesic activity of LAS 1 mg was present 20, 80 and 140 minutes after the icv injection (licking time significantly reduced compared to the control group); it disappeared after 200 minutes.

When comparing the degree of the analgesia obtained by icv LAS 1 mg to that obtained by icv morphine, the latter was significantly more powerful in suppressing the nociceptive behaviour.

No evident side effects or complications occurred following icv injections.

Discussion

In '87 a report was published by French authors[3] claiming remarkable analgesia following intrathecal injection of LAS in 60 patients. The rationale for injecting such a drug was to reduce the synthesis of pain mediators such as PGF2 at the spinal level[4].

Our clinical experience was discouraging: in 6 patients complaining of persistent side effects after intrathecal morphine we injected 125–1000 mg of LAS. Only one patient reported 70% of analgesia lasting for 60 hours. No analgesic effect of clinical usefulness was achieved in the remaining 5 patients. Our experimental study showed that icv LAS at high doses was able to significantly modify the nociceptive behaviour in mice and for a relatively short period of time (less than 200 minutes). No effect was evident at lower dosage. Furthermore, the analgesic effect of LAS 1 mg was significantly less powerful than that of icv morphine. The administration of LAS was not followed by any obvious side effects in mice; however, the intrathecal administration of LAS in man was accompanied by serious side effects (vomiting, sonnolence, monoparesis) in 4 of our 6 patients, and similar complications are reported in literature[3].

On the basis of our clinical and animal experience we stopped using LAS into the CSF for pain control.

Acknowledgements

Supported by MPI 60%.

Thanks are due to Prof. S. Ferri and Dr. S. Candeletti (Institute of Pharmacology, University of Bologna) for methodological suggestions.

References

1. Devoghel JC (1983) Small intrathecal doses of acetylsalicylate relieve intractable pain in man. J Int Med Res 11: 90–91
2. Murray CW, Porreca F, Cowan A (1988) Methodological refinements to the mouse paw Formalin test. An animal model of tonic pain. J Pharm Meth 20: 175–186
3. Pellerin M, Hardy F, Abergel A, Boule D, Palacci JH, Babinet P, Wingtin LNG, Glowinski J, Amiot JF, Mechali D, Colbert N, Starkman M (1987) Douleur chronique rebelle des cancéreux. Intéret de l'injection intrarachidienne d'acétylsalicylate de lysine. La Presse Med 30: 1465–1467
4. Yaksh TL (1982) Central and peripherical mechanisms for the antialgesic action of acetylsalicyclic acid. In: Barnett JJ, Mustard JF (eds) New uses for an old drug. Raven Press, New York, pp 137–158

Correspondence: Prof M. Meglio, Istituto di Neurochirurgia, Università Cattolica, lg. A. Gemelli 8, I-00168 Roma, Italy.

Open Stereotactic Neurosurgery

Acta Neurochirurgica, Suppl. 52, 9–12 (1991)

Open Stereotactic Surgery

E. Hitchcock

Department of Neurosurgery, University of Birmingham, West Midlands, UK

Summary

Open Stereotactic Surgery [OSS] may be defined as the use of precise stereotactic techniques to facilitate conventional neurosurgical procedures.

The field has expanded in recent years particularly in the areas of imaging, instrumentation and co-ordinate transfer.

The factors influencing the developments are explored.

Keywords: Stereotactic; Craniotomy.

One of the most profound changes taking place in neurosurgery and in surgery in general has been the replacement of large operative procedures with comparatively minor percutaneous or endoscopic ones. It has been particularly dramatic in neurosurgery where many previously open procedures performed under general anaesthesia are executed more precisely, more safely and more quickly under local anaesthesia. It is obvious however that not all conditions can be treated thus, and the second most important revolution has been the use of these precise stereotactic techniques to facilitate formal craniotomy and tumour extirpation, for which the term "open stereotactic surgery" has been coined[1]. The development of modern imaging has encouraged better use of the revelation of hidden features and their position in intracranial space.

Riechert (1980)[7] was one of the first to use stereotactic apparatus for conventional neurosurgical operations largely for trans-sphenoidal hypophysectomy with the operative microscope. A true open stereotactic technique was used for the extraction of intracerebral foreign bodies and permitted small craniotomies. Several workers were encouraged to use the stereotactic technique for localisation of foreign bodies probably because the majority were sufficiently opaque to enable precise localisation. Small fragments can be removed through a burr hole without using craniotomy and do not qualify for the term open stereotactic surgery[2]. This should be reserved for procedures using craniotomy although the term stereotactic craniotomy does not cover other important aspects such as the use of specific stereotactic instrumentation. A true open stereotactic procedure was used by Zamskaya[10] in excising epileptic focci. Riechert[7] proved most original in his approach to "central angiomas" and pointed to the advantages of stereotaxy in finding the often elusive microangiomas and relating their site to surrounding important structures. I have used the stereotactic technique to locate the nidus or the arterial feeders to large arteriovenous malformations although stereotactic irradiation is now preferred.

The development of open stereotactic surgery has proceeded in three main areas: steteotactic imaging, stereotactic instrumentation and stereotactic co-ordinate transfer. *Stereotactic imaging* has been dealt with exhaustively over the past decade and it is only necessary to record that open stereotactic surgery (OSS) has used a variety of image systems. *Straight x-rays* are invaluable in targeting high density FBs such as metal which produce gross artifact in CT and MRI but the use of straight x-rays are subordinate to *CT scanning* which is still the most common and useful stereotactic imaging modality. It is quick and cheap but its simple images do not support complex pathological analysis. MRI provides superb pictures of normal structures but unhappily has not lived up to its promise of revealing the character of intrinsic tumour and we cannot yet reliably distinguish oedema, oedematous tumour or tumour.

Stereotactic instrument. There are also special problems associated with these computerised images related to the interface between image and stereotactic instrument. High atomic weight substances have huge CT signals and thus the stereotactic instrument itself may produce considerable artifact. One of the most familiar of these is the cross produced by four steel pins, the number of bar artifacts produced being directly related to the number of pins. The instrument base itself produces considerable artifact and in MRI great distortion. This can be avoided by using non-metallic material like wood or certain plastics and reduced by using non-ferrous material such as aluminium. The use of fiducals allows placement of the stereotactic base below the scanning level and the less artifactual fiducals permit mathematical derivations of target position.

To be effective the stereotactic base must be low profiled and many popular models are gradually removing their cubic and artifactual structures to gain the low profiles favoured by other instruments (Figs. 1 and 2). Another advantage of a low base profile is that the apparatus is light, stable and free of extraneous projections such as fixation posts. This means that the patient may move freely and painlessly whilst wearing the apparatus permitting chronic wear for days if needed; most importantly it clears the head of obstructions to craniotomy. There is certainly some restriction compared to conventional craniotomy but the precise localisation of the mass means that very much smaller exposures are needed. It should be possible to visually check that the target and the trajectory are "sensible" (Fig. 3). Computers certainly give accuracy but can break down and it is dangerous to have to rely absolutely upon them. Indeed the important thing to remember about all forms of

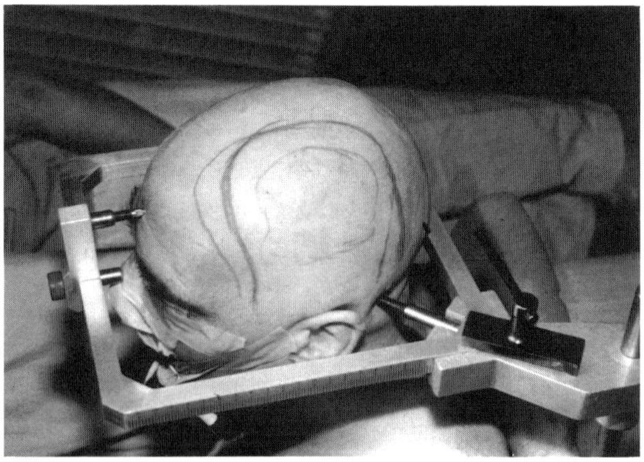

Fig. 1. The stereotactic square has a low profile which permits wide exposure of the skull

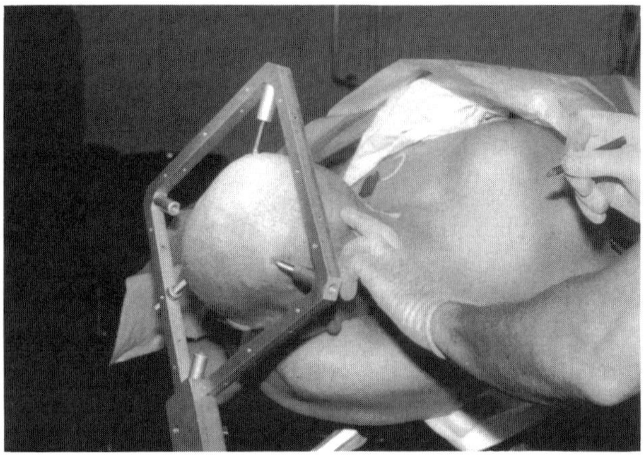

Fig. 2. A low profile square facilitates infratentorial procedures as well as supratentorial

stereotaxy is that complexity is a dangerous luxury. Unless dedicated CT's or substantial CT time is made available specifically for stereotactic use the stereotactic base will be contaminated. It must be possible therefore to clean and sterilise the base while still on the patients head and to be able to do this confidently immediately pre-operatively.

The application of CT imaging to open stereotactic surgery was soon recognised and many centres including my own were using stereotactic techniques as an aid to precise localised craniotomy in lesion identification. Later in the 1980's new instrumentation was developed specifically designed for open stereotactic procedures[1,3,4,6,8].

In the last few years interest in open stereotactic surgery increased enormously as the advantages became obvious to those who are not primarily stereotactic neurosurgeons and there is hardly a stereotactic instrument that has not been modified and then extolled as ideal for open stereotactic surgery[5].

Great morbidity and mortality is associated with attempts to remove intracranial masses from certain sites such as deep basal nuclei and close to the ventricles. The precise localisation possible for stereotaxy allows the surgeon to go directly to the mass despite the presence of the common peritumoural oedema which otherwise makes localisation hazardous. Additionally because of this precision small cortical incisions can be planned through the least functionally important areas via small craniotomies. The simplicity of some systems is such that many of these procedures can be performed under local anaesthesia and the ability of modern stereo imaging techniques to integrate stereotactic angiograms into

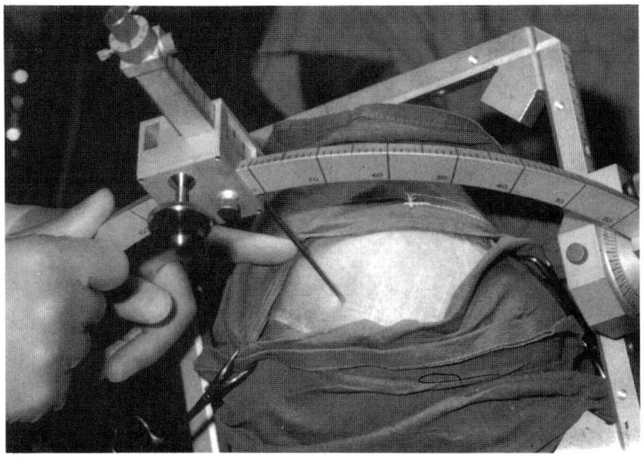

Fig. 3. The guiding probe or cannula can be seen to be correctly aligned

the image gives a further safety factor in avoiding damage.

Although special instrumentation has been developed for open stereotactic surgery they are invariably expensive. Many of the standard stereotactic apparatus can be used for open technique with no or minimal modification. The ideal instrument for open stereotactic surgery must of course be accurate and image adaptable. Kelly and others[5,9] have provided beautiful images using sophisticated computer techniques but not without expense. The integration of 3-D images into the stereotactic apparatus is expensive. Provided the approximate tumour volume and the exact target co-ordinates can be programmed, possibly with angiographic integration, the simplest localisations and demonstrations of tumours is usually sufficient.

Stereotactic co-ordinate transfer. For most deep lesions the most that is required is the target co-ordinate; depending on the size of the tumour the target will be the most superficial point or commonly the centre of the mass. The simplest imaging system is therefore acceptable. Either the stereotactic base itself is attached to the imaging system and isocentered or the conventional fidical system with an unfixed stereotactic instrument is fixed to the patient's head the target point and co-ordinates are calculated by computer. An attractive alternative is to establish the target co-ordinates by some intermediate device which can be subsequently integrated with the main stereotactic instrument. Such a device has many advantages not the least of which is the ability to allow an interval between imaging and operation. It is helpful too whilst performing the procedure to be able to maintain the three dimensional orientation either by the use of stereotactic microscopes or retractors, projection light sources or in the case of the Kelly device the integration of the microscope with the CT scan and stereotactic instrument.

There is good evidence that the removal of a single brain metastasis substantially improves a patients quality and quantity of life. Certain metastases however are so placed that their identification and removal by conventional methods may have a high morbidity and mortality; it is here that open stereotactic excision is most successful and I have used this method for both supratentorial and infratentorial tumours. Excluding patients where the stereotactic base and guiding devices have been used to simply locate the lesion about one third of cases are metastasis and one third are deep seated gliomas. I have also used this technique for benign lesions such as arteriovenous malformations and meningiomas. In the small and especially in the superficial lesions it has been possible to perform the whole procedure under local anaesthesia.

Opponents of stereotactic procedures in general will complain that undue complexity is introduced to what is a straight-forward and conventional neurosurgery. However my experience has been that stereotactic localisation itself gives considerable advantages and can shorten the operative time considerably. However stereotactic localisation must be reasonably quick and if there is much time added to the operating procedure in localising the lesion it will not continue to be popular and instead techniques such as ultrasound localisation will be adopted as providing sufficient aids in localisation.

The method used in my department has developed over ten years or more and has shown itself to be simple, safe, accurate and increasingly popular in terms of patient referral. Essentially the technique is the application of the flat profile stereotactic square which takes five minutes. The stereotactic scanning can be as simple (10 minutes) or as complex (multiple re-formation 20 minutes) as the surgeon wishes. Because the stereotactic square is isocentred to the CT scan all measurements and calculations appear on the CT console using the CT machine internal computer. The patient is then taken to the operating theatre with the co-ordinates and fixed to the operating table by a simple attachment that attaches to the Mayfield head holder.

For simple localisation it is sufficient to use a probe or biopsy cannula; either a planned trajectory can be chosen or from direct observation a suitable trajectory chosen to avoid vulnerable areas and make the shortest tract. For small lesions a simple aiming tube can be attached to the arc through which the beam of an operating microscope can be directed and the procedure accomplished microsurgically, adjusting the microscope to fit the inclination of the tube as required. Alternatively brain retractors are used for larger lesions conveniently fixed to the stereotactic base itself together with other attachments useful for conventional microsurgery. The fact that the Society has chosen to give one whole session up to open stereotactic surgery is evidence of the increasing importance of this expanding field which is likely to have as major an effect in conventional neurosurgery as it has interest in stereotactic societies.

References

1. Hitchcock ER (1985) Open stereotactic excisional surgery. Appl Neurophysiol 48: 86–88
2. Hitchcock E, Cowie R (1982) Stereotactic removal of intracranial foreign bodies: review and case report. Injury 14: 471–475
3. Jacques S, Sheldon H, McCann GD, Freshwater DB, Rand R (1980) Computerized three dimensional stereotaxis removal of small central nervous system lesions in patients. J Neurosurg 53: 816–820
4. Kelly PJ, Goess SJ, Kall BA (1988) Evolution of contemporary instrumentation for computer-assisted stereotactic surgery. Surg Neurol 30: 204–215
5. Moore MR, Black P McL, Ellenbogen R, Gall CM, Eldridge E (1989) Stereotactic craniotomy: Methods and results using the Brown and Roberts-Wells stereotactic frame. Neurosurgery 25 (4): 572–578
6. Patel AA (1987) Stereotactic excision of deep brain lesions using probe guided brain retractor. Acta Neurochir (Wien) 87: 50–152
7. Riechert T (1980) Stereotactic brain operations: Methods, clinical aspects, indications. Hans-Huber, Berne, Stuttgart, Vienna pp 1–387
8. Sheldon EH, McLann G, Jacques S *et al* (1980) Development of a computerized macrostereotaxis method for localisastion and removal of minute CNS lesions under direct 3-D vision: Technical report. J Neurosurg 52: 21–27
9. Zamorans L, Martinez-Coll A, Dujorny (1989) Transposition of image-defined trajectories into arc-quadrant centred stereotactic systems. Acta Neurochir (Wien) [Suppl 1] 46: 109–111
10. Zamskaya AG, Garmeshor Ju A, Ryabukha NP (1976) Application with classical craniotomy in the treatment of focal epilepsy. Acta Neurochir (Wien) [Suppl] 23: 147–151

Correspondence: Prof. Dr. E. Hitchcock, Department of Neurosurgery, University of Birmingham, Midland Centre for Neurosurgery and Neurology, Holly Lane, Smethwick, West Midlands, B67 7JX, UK.

Acta Neurochirurgica, Suppl. 52, 13–14 (1991)

Open Stereotactic Neurosurgery: 57 Cases

F. Giunta and **G. Marini**

Neurosurgery, University of Brescia, Spedali Civili, Brescia, Italy

Summary

The two main neurosurgical tools are the operative microscope and stereotactic apparatus. The operative microscope is essential in cisternal or ventricular surgery and the stereotactic apparatus is essential in approaching intracerebral lesions. Both given their best performance when the one aids the other. Small convexity lesions are best approach with stereotactic aid, and excellent microsurgical intracerebral lesions can be debulked with the operative microscope.

Malignant tumours pursue their inevitable course but slow growing tumours and angiomas may have long survival even with one subtotal removal. The major problem in removing slow-growing tumors is the difficulty in distinguishing tumour from normal brain, but the stereotactic guide is useful in delimitating tumour volume.

The results in 57 cases are described.

Keywords: Open stereotactic neurosurgery; results.

Introduction

In this CT era many brain lesions can be visualized and their site and extension exactly displayed. The stereotactic instrument is the only appropriate surgical instrument for many and an histopathological diagnosis was obtained in 96%. Open surgery with a stereotactic guide was developed not only to reach the lesion but to estimate the spatial extension of the lesion. In Open stereotactic Surgery a craniotomy is performed to remove under direct vision a solid brain lesion reached with a stereotactic guide and with stereotactic spatial deliniation. Stereotaxis allows precise localization and volume identification of the lesion visualized from CT scans and consequently protects the perilesional brain from surgical trauma.

The stereotactic approach is advised for the management of deep brain lesions by many authors[1]–12, but many small cortical or subcortical lesions are also suitable.

Material and Methods

From 1983 to 1989 we performed 57 open stereotactic approaches to brain expansive lesions. The indications for open stereotactic procedure were removal of small lesions in cortical subcortical areas mainly in eloquent regions (Roland, Broca, Wernike and Calcarina) and deep central Regions (basal ganglia, internal capsula and thalamus). 30 were male and 25 female. Age ranged from 5 to 67 years (average 37). The site of the 57 surgical procedures was: 18 eloquent areas, 22 non eloquent areas, 17 central [basal ganglia, internal capsule, thalamus]. The surgical procedure combined stereotactic and microsurgical techniques. After shaving the hair the stereotactic frame is applied to the scale. CT scans are used to calculate stereotactic coordinates. Often a 1″ or 2″ trephine was used for craniotomy. Using a stereotactically orientated needle as a guide, the tumour is reached and removed. Transparent and malleable brain retractors are used to follow the stereotactic needle to the target and microscopy or endoscopy used to visualize the tumour which is removed with the sucker or forceps around the tip of the stereotactic needle. Bipolar coagulation is used for haemostasis. It is very important, especially in benign tumours, that the stereotactic needle stays on the target during the surgery because the volume of the tumour removed is calculated around it. The surgical approach from cortex to deep brain tumours has a conic shape and a small corticotomy (1 cm) is sufficient to remove any tumour with minimal brain trauma. If the tumour tissue cannot be distinguished from normal brain, an ideal stereotactic reconstruction of the tumour volume is performed by calculating the CT diameters of the lesion around the trajectory of the stereotactic needle.

Result

Histology showed: 23 fast-growing tumours (13 metastases, 3 glioblastomas, one AIDS pathology, 6 anaplastic astrocytoma, (1 anaplastic oligodendroglioma), 30 slow-growing tumours (6 pilocytic a., 10 fibrillary, a., 4 protoplasmic a., 5 gemistocytuc a., 3 oligodendrogliomas, 1 meningioma, 1 neurofibroma) and 4 no-tumour (3 cryptic angioma, 1 small periventricular avm).

Table 1. *Site, Number of Patients, Histopathology and Surgical Outcome in 57 Open Stereotactic Surgery*

Site	No. Pat.	Histology	Surgical Outcome
Eloquent areas	18	6 slow growing astrocytoma	2 worse but recovered
		1 small meningioma (1 cm)	
		1 fast growing astrocytoma	
		7 metastases	
		3 cryptic angioma	
Deep subcortical	22	12 slow growing astrocytoma	1 worse
		4 fast growing astrocytoma	1 death, 2 worse
		5 metastases	
		1 periventricular AVM	
Central regions	17	10 slow growing astrocytoma	
		1 neurofibroma	
		5 fast growing astrocytoma	1 worse
		1 metastases	

Central regions are: basal ganglia, internal capsula and thalamus

Total removal was possible in well delimited lesions and usually all pathological tissues seen was removed. When pathological tissue was difficult to recognize volumes similar to those observed in CT were removed. All patients with benign tumour (53%) are living and seizures are well controlled in all but two. There was one surgical death (1.9%) in a patient with an anaplastic astrocytoma; 6 patients (11.5%) developed neurological deterioration but two recovered. (Table 1).

References

1. Hariz KI, Fodstad H (1987) Stereotactic localization of small subcortical tumour for open surgery. Surg Neurol 28: 345–350
2. Hitchcock ER (1985) Open stereotactic excisional surgery. Appl Neurophysiol 48: 86–88
3. Kall BA, Kelly PJ, Goerss SJ (1985) Interactive stereotactic surgical system for removal of intracranial tumors utilizing the CO_2 laser and CT-derived database. IEEE Trans Biomed Eng 32: 112–116
4. Kelly PJ, Alker GJ, Goerss SJ (1982) Computer-assisted stereotactic microsurgery for the treatment of intracranial neoplasms. Neurosurgery 10: 324–331
5. Kelly PJ, Kall BA, Goerss SJ (1983) Stereotactic CT scanning for the biopsy of intracranial lesions and functional neurosurgery. Appl Neurophysiol 46: 193–199
6. Kelly PJ, Kall BA, Goerss SJ (1987) Computer interactive stereotactic resection of deep-seated and centrally located intra-axial brain lesions. Appl Neurophysiol 50: 107–113
7. McGirr SJ, Kelly PJ, Scheithauer BW (1987) Stereotactic resection of juvenile pilocytic astrocytoma of the thalamus and basal ganglia. Neurosurgery 20: 447–452
8. Mitchem HL (1984) A CT guided stereotactic apparatus: New approach to biopsy and removal of brain tumors. J Neurosurg Nurs 16: 231–236
9. Patil AA (1987) Stereotactic excision of deep brain lesions using probe guided brain retractor. Acta Neurochir (Wien) 87: 150–152
10. Rougier A, Loiseau P, Rivel J, Cohadon F, Orgogozo JM (1984) Epilepsies partielles de l'adolescene avec anomalies tomodensitometriques, reaction astrocytaire localisee, evolution spontanement regressive. Rev Neurol (Paris) 140: 171–178
11. Shelden CH, Jacques S, McCann G (1982) The Shelden CT-based microneurosurgical stereotactic system: Its application to CNS pathology. Appl Neurophysiol 45: 341–346
12. Steude AU, Hamburger C (1987) Pre-operative stereotactic localization of cerebral tumours: A new tool to improve microsurgical tumor removal. Appl Neurophysiol 50: 241–242

Correspondence: F. Giunta, Neurosurgery, University of Brescia, Şpedali Çivili, Brescia, Italy.

Acta Neurochirurgica, Suppl. 52, 15–18 (1991)

Stereotactic Open Craniotomy and Laser Resection of Brain Tumours A Five Years Experience.

J. Eiras, J. Alberdi, L.I. Carcavilla, J. Gomez, and **J. Cantero**

Neurosurgical Regional Service, Hospital "Miguel Servet", Zaragoza, Spain

Summary

In 23 cases of deep-seated brain tumours stereotactically guided laser vaporization has been done, using a 60 watts CO_2 laser. The experiences and results of the 18 first cases with a follow-up of 10 months to 5 years are presented. The technique is described.

Keywords: Brain tumour; CO_2 laser vaporization; stereotactic guidance; results.

Introduction

Surgical treatment of deep-seated tumours, has been associated with high morbidity and incomplete removals. It is especially true with small neoplasms in the subcortical white matter due to difficulties in localization, poor spatial orientation and the unclear delineation of the neoplastic tissue boundaries.

The introduction of stereotactic techniques to guide the open surgical procedures when dealing with small and deep-seated lesions is quite old[13,14], but in recent years it has been associated with microsurgical techniques and CT-compatible stereotactic frames[1,2,3,11,14]. More sophisticated technical advances include the vaporization of the tumour with lasers,[4,6] determination of volume and shape with computers, data acquisition from the MRI[7,12,15] and the use of endoscopy or ultrasounds in the surgical field[1,4,15].

In the present paper, we report our experience, current methodology and results obtained in eighteen cases of intracerebral small deep-seated tumours, treated with a 60 watts CO_2 laser vaporization (Sharplan Ind.) stereotactically guided with the data from CT and MRI.

Material and Methods

A. Surgical Procedure

Under local anesthesia a CT-compatible stereotactic frame built in plastic material is fixed to the patient's skull by three aluminium alloy screws. The frame is a third prototype derived from a Riechert-Mundinger device and is also MRI compatible. Fiducial marks in the CT scan are obtained from metallic wires with a "N" disposition included in a plastic hollow cylinder as in other stereotactical systems (Fig. 1). The marks used for the MRI study are obtained from 3 mm paraffin-filled tubes. The X, Y and Z, coordinates of the target point, other reference points, trajectory, volume and shape of the tumour are calculated by computer and transferred to a phantom. The patient, is then anaethetized in the operating room.

Our guide holder system permits without new calculations-biopsies in an area of 2.5 cms radius around the initial trajectory, changes of the biopsy cannula for an endoscope or the adaptation of cylindrical brain retractors.

A craniotomy with a 3–4 cm of diameter is centered around the entry point. The CO_2 laser, coupled with the microscope, is moved to the operating field and the He-Ne aiming beam of the laser is aligned in the biopsy-cannula direction. The microscope arms are strongly fixed in order to avoid deviations in the trajectory to the target point.

A linear corticotomy is performed using a mean power of 4 watts, moderately defocussed and in continuous mode. Small retractors can be used manually to spread the brain incision. We have developed a set of cylindrical plastic and metallic retractors of various lengths and diameters which fits into the guide holder. To get down into the tumour, a cannula with a inflatable ballon in the tip is placed in the "mouth" of the cylindrical retractors in order to dilate the wound and avoid damage in the subcortical white matter (Fig. 2). The wound depth can be read on the retractors or assessed by replacing the cannula or by biplane radiology. Such corticotomy can be also done in a standard way or guided by a plastic catheter down to the tumour's surface.

The tumour surface is coagulated with 3–5 watts and its core is vaporized with powers of 10 to 30 watts. In hypervascularized tumours, the superpulsed mode use avoids the oozing usually seen with the CO_2 laser. The tubular retractors can be moved to follow

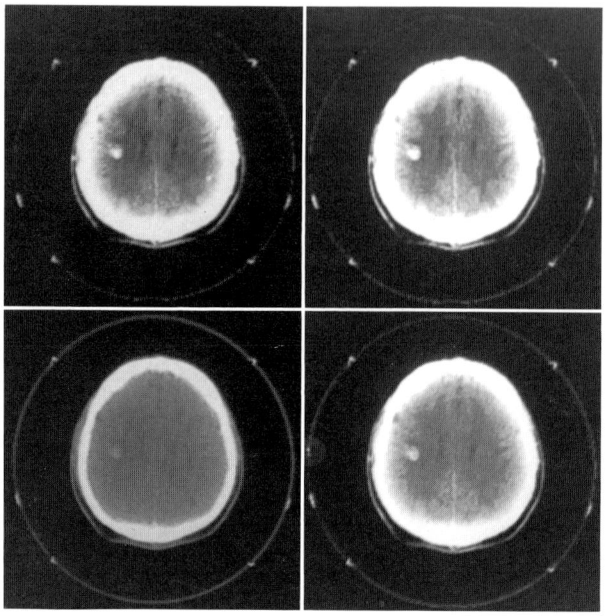

a

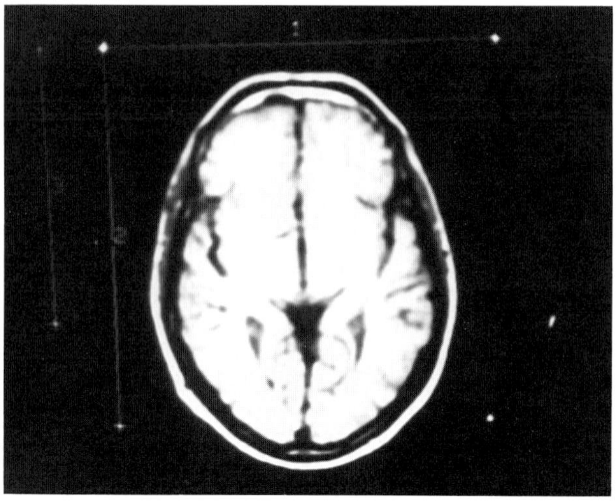

b

Fig. 1. (a) CT slice with the stereotactic frame and localization system in a case of subcortical tumour. The metallic marks engraved in the plastic hollow cylinder gives six fine reference points. (b) MRI slice with the stereotactic frame. The fiducials are obtained from 3 mm. paraffin filled tubes

the irregular borders of the tumour but a return to the target point is always possible by centering the He-Ne beam in the microscope photographic reticula, replacing the biopsy cannula or using biplane radiological facilities.

In cystic lesions an endoscope can be introduced through a burr hole, replacing the cannula, to visualize the lesion, to preform a biopsy or to vaporize the tumour by coupling with the CO_2 laser arm. This technique was used in two of our patients.

B. Clinical Material

Since 1985, 23 patients have been operated on with this technique, though only the first 18 with a follow up ranging from 5 year to 10 months will be discussed in this paper.

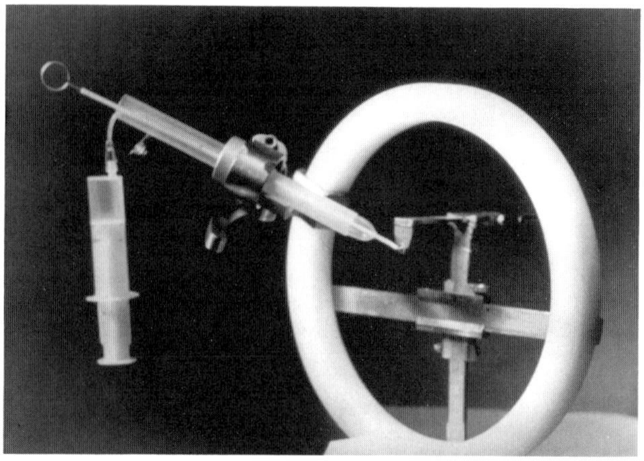

Fig. 2. Guide holder system attached to the phantom ring. A plastic tubular retractor is aimed at the target point. An inflatable catheter can be seen inside the retractor

There were 11 men and 7 women, with ages ranging from 11 to 64 years. Initial symptoms were convulsive seizures in 9, in 4 progressive intracranial hypertension due to obstructive hydrocephalus, in 4 hemiparesis and in 1 case subarachnoid haemorrhage.

In every case the CT and MRI demonstrated a deeply placed expansive process with size ranging from 1 × 1 × 1 to 3 × 5 × 4 cms, mean size 3 × 2 × 3 cms. The mean estimated volume was 16.4 c.c. In 12 cases the tumour was in the dominant hemisphere, in 3 it was medially placed and in 3 cases it was located in the non dominant side.

The preoperative rediological assessment suggested a low grade astrocytoma in 10 cases.

Results

No neurological deficit appeared after the surgical procedure in 11 patients, in 5 cases mild and transient motor weakness was detected, in 2 cases transient speech disturbance and in one case of left parieto-occipital astrocytoma a visual field defect was the only neurological sequela. No patient died as a result of the surgical intervention.

The accuracy of the surgical resection was evaluated as "high" when the tumour removal was complete or over 80% of the presumed preoperative volume, "medium" when it was over 50% and "minimal" when it was under 50%. In 16 cases the precision was high, in 2 medium and minimal in none.

Tolerance to the surgical trauma was evaluated in relation to postoperative complaints, bed rest time and days of hospital stay. It was considered "very good" in 15 cases, "normal" or similar to a conventional procedure in 2 and "bad" in 1 patient of 61 years with a III ventricle astrocytoma.

The final pathological diagnosis was in 10 cases astrocytomata (7 fibrilary, 3 grades II-III) in 2 cases ependymoma, 2 cases metastasis (kidney and digestive tract), 1 case cavernoma, 1 case ependymal cyst, 1 case craniopharngioma and 1 case of meningioma of the lateral ventricle of the dominant hemisphere.

Discussion

Stereotactic craniotomy is widely accepted as a precise system to reach deep and small intracerebral targets into the brain. On the other hand, the CO_2 laser provides a hands-off method fordestroying neoplasic tissue. The conjunction of both methods allows the neurosurgeon to deal with small and deep seated tumours with great accuracy and minimal neurological deficits[4,5,6,8,10].

Inherent *advantages in the stereotactic technique* are:
1.-Maximal accuracy in determining the place, shape and volume of the lesion.
2.-Possibility of integrating CT, MRI and DA. Data.
3.-Selection of the least traumatic point for corticotomy and of the angles to reach the tumour.
4.-The working channel is unique and accurate to the target point.
5.-The shape of the working window can be superimposed on the shape of the mass in every slice.
6.-Spatial orientation is possible in every step of the resection[7,12,15].

Advantages derived from the Co_2 laser are:
1.-Possibility of working through a minimal approach unsuitable for bulky instruments.
2.-Minimal trauma to surrounding tissue by using a hand-off technique.
3.-Minimizes haemorrhage.

All these advantages have been widely discussed after the pioneering work of Kelly et al. However some *draw backs* should be exposed:
1.-The stereotactic procedure is time-consuming. Although the computerized data treatment can be done in minutes, gathering images from the CT. NMR and DA requires many hours and the coordination of several departments in the hospital. In some institutions the procedure is performed in separate sessions.
2.-The accuracy of some MRI images is uncertain.
3.-A perfect cylindrical retractor which avoid trauma to the subcortical white matter requires development.
4.-The ash produced by the CO_2 laser may interfere, with the visualization of the clevage plane between tumour and normal tissue.
5.-Fluid leakage from cysts or ventrices may change the spatial situation of the tumour diminishing accuracy.
6.-With malignant tumours the technique has superiority over convenctional microsurgical procedures[9,10].

Although the advantages outweigh the disadvantages, the afore mentioned considerations has limited our technique to small benign, deep seated tumours in functional areas or in the dominant hemisphere. Only 18 of 533 brain tumours treated in the same period were operated on with this technique.

The long duration and the high cost of the procedure are the only real disadvantages in relation to the conventional neurosurgical method. The accuracy lesser surgical trauma and low risk of the stereotactic procedure plus the increasingly frequent diagnosis of small intracerebral masses will give to this method a great future.

References

1. Appuzzo MLJ, Sabshin JL (1983) Computed tomographic guidance stereotaxis in the management of intracerebral mass lesions. Neurosurgery 12: 277–285
2. Boethius J, Bergström M, Greitz T (1980) Stereotactic computerized tomography with a GE 8800 scanner. J Neurosurg 52: 794–800
3. Brown RA (1979) A computerized tomography-computer graphics approachtostereotaxic localization. J Neurosurg 50: 715–720
4. Eiras J, Carcavilla L, Gomez-Perun J, Alberdi J (1987) CO_2 laser vaporization of deep seated tumors with a CT directed stereotaxic system. Abstract book. 8th European Congress of Neurosurgery. Barcelona 6–11 September
5. Hitchcock ER (1985) Open Stereotactic excisional Surgery. Appl Neurophysical 48: 86–88
6. Kelly PJ, Alker GJ Junior (1981) A stereotactic approach to deep seated CNS neoplasms using the carbon dioxide laser. Surg Neurol 15: 331–334
7. Kelly PJ, Kall BA, Goerss SJ (1984) Transposition of volumetric information derived from C.T. scanning into stereotactic space. Surg Neurol 21: 465–471
8. Kelly PJ, Kall BA, Goerss J (1986) Computed-assisted stereotactic resection of posterior fossa lesions. Surg Neurol 25: 530–534
9. Kelly PJ, Kall BA, Goerss SJ (1988) Results of computed topmography-based computer-assisted stereotactic resection of metastatic intracranial tumours. Neurosurgery 22(1): 7–18
10. Kelly PJ (1988) Glial neoplasms: Conventional and stereotactic applications. In: Cerullo LJ (ed) Applications of Lasers in Neurosurgery Ch.7 Year Book Med. Publishers Inc. Chicago, London, Boca Raton pp 82–99
11. Koslow M, Abele MG, Griffith RC, Mair GA, Chase NE (1981) Stereotactic surgical system controlled by computed tomography. Neurosurgery 8: 72–82
12. Peters TM, Clark JA, Pike GB, Henri C, Collins L, Leksell D, Jeppsson O (1989) Stereotactic neurosurgery planning on a personal-computer-based work station. J Digital Imaging 2(2): 75–81

13. Riechert T, Mundinger F (1964) Combined stereotaxic operation for treatment of deep seated angiomas and aneurysms. J Neurosurg, 21: 358–363
14. Shelden CH, McCann G, Jaques S, Lutes HR, Frazier RE, Katz R, Kuki R (1980) Development of a computerized microstereotaxic method for localization and removal of minute CNS lesions under direct 3-D vision. Technical report. J Neurosurg 52: 21–27
15. Zamorano L, Dujovny M, Malik G, Mehta B (1988) Transposition of MRI data into multiplanar 130 CT stereotaxis. Abstract book. 8th Meeting of the European Society for Stereotactic and Functional Neurosurgery, Budapest, June 1–3

Correspondence: J. Eiras, Jefe Servicio Neurocirugia, Hospital "Miguel Servet", E-50009 Zaragoza, Spain.

Acta Neurochirurgica, Suppl. 52, 19–21 (1991)

Deep Seated Cerebral Lesion Removal, Guided by Volumetric Rendering of Morphological Data, Stereotactically Acquired Clinical Results and Technical Considerations

C. Giorgi, E. Ongania, S.D. Casolino, D. Riva[1]**, G. Cella, A. Franzini,** and **G. Broggi**

Departments of Neurosurgery and [1]Child Neurology, Istituto Neurologico "C. Besta", Milano, Italy

Summary

The theoretical advantages of microsurgery guided by volumetric reconstruction of anatomy in stereotactic space, compared to traditional technique are discussed. Preliminary clinical results in 30 cases and technical considerations, concerning future developments, are presented.

Keywords: Brain tumours; subcortical; stereotactical removal; results.

Introduction

A growing interest in the development of instrumentation for guided microsurgery has been recorded[1,3,5,6,7] after the introduction of stereotaxy in the domain of open surgery[4].

The solutions usually derive from a straightforward translation of stereotactic methods and instruments into open surgery, and consist of a spatial description of a target point within the lesion volume, which is reached by means of aiming tools. Such devices may vary from a simple plastic tube, inserted in the cerebral parenchyma along the selected trajectory, or other less invasive methods (laser light), to guide the surgeon in approaching the lesion.

All these methods, based on the identification of a target on stereotactically acquired CT or MRI images, provide definitive advantages over "traditional" procedures, in the surgery of subcortical lesions. These lesions can also be reached with the aid of intra-operative echography but a stereotactic guide offers advantages compared to the use of hand-held echographic probe in locating subcortical lesions: it allows for the selection of a trajectory of approach that takes into consideration the functional relevance of the incised cortex. The deeper the lesion, the greater the choice of possible approach trajectories: an echographic image gives the surgeon the position of a lesion in the direction orthogonal to the surface, while the proper use of neuroanatomical imaging reconstruction and stereotactic instrumentation assists the surgeon in finding the most suitable "functional" trajectory. Furthermore, the integration of stereotactic angiography with MRI and CT data adds to the safety of the chosen surgical approach.

From a practical point of view, however, these theoretical advantages are deminished by the burden of "additional preparation", such as special draping, acquisition of images under stereotactic conditions, target identification, and calculation of the trajectory, when compared to the straightforward use of an echographic probe. This is probably the single most important reason why the development of surgical instrumentation for guided removal of cerebral lesions is carried out at a slow pace, when compared to the potential improvement of the practice of neurosurgery that could derive from it.

Our experience in the field of guided neurosurgery dates back to the summer of 1987. Acquisition of MRI and CT under stereotactic conditions and volumetric reconstruction of the lesion and surrounding structures have been performed in all 30 cases, using a PC based graphic workstation and imaging handling software, developed at our Institution. The surgical approach has been simulated on a graphic monitor, and the chosen trajectory has been translated in the operative space, using commercially available stereotactic frames. The method has already been described

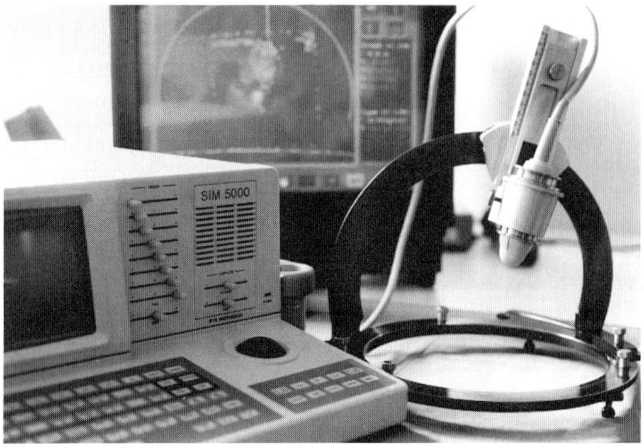

Fig. 1. Stereotactic echographic apparatus, showing a 5.5 Mhz probe mounted on a stereotactic frame. Images are processed by a surgical graphic console

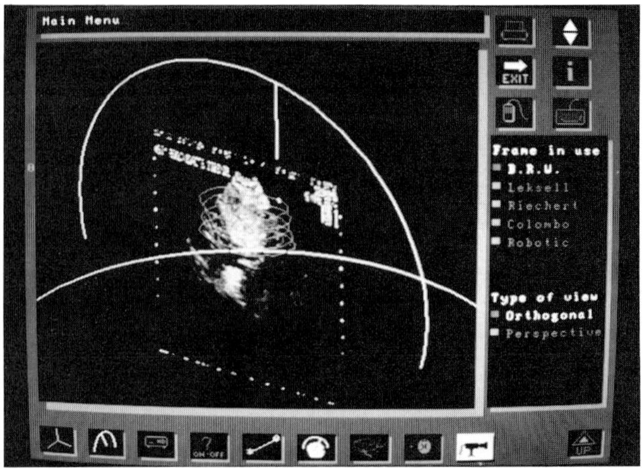

Fig. 2. An echographic image displayed on the graphic reconstruction of a cerebral glioma, outlined from stereotactically acquired CT images. Satisfactory superimposition of the contrast-enhanced lesion within the hypodense area is obtained

elsewhere[2]. Recently, the procedure has been integrated with the stereotactic acquisition of echographic images, obtained at the beginning and during consecutive phases of the procedure (Figs. 1 and 2). The probe is mounted on the stereotactic frame; the image plane is known and can be displayed by the graphic monitor onto the volumetric reconstruction of the lesion, outlined from MRI or CT images. The graphic

Table 1.

Age Sex	Site	Lesion Removal		Outcome	F.UP
17F	DT + BG	Low grade astrocyt.	70%	improved	1,5yr
35F	DP	Oligodendroglioma	70%	improved	2yr
58F	DT + BG	Glioblastoma	75%	improved	1yr
17M	BG	Low grade astrocyt.	100%	normal	2yr
40M	DP	AVM	100%	normal	1.5yr–2P.
52F	BG	Oligoastrocytoma	50%	unchanged	2yr
48M	BG	Glioblastoma	80%	death	
45F	BG	Glioblastoma	50%	improved	1yr
32M	DP	Low grade astrocyt.	100%	normal	15yr
50M	P	Metastatic	100%	improved	6mo
23F	BG.	Glioblastoma	50%	improved	1yr
25M	III v.	Mal. Teratoma	95%	improved	2mo–rec.
6M	BG	Subep. astrocyt.	90%	improved	1yr
28F	i.v.	Oligodendroglioma	100%	normal	1.5yr
14F	BG	Pilocytic astrocyt.	100%	normal	1yr
23M	BG	Oligoastrocyt.	100%	improved	1yr–2P.
25M	BG	Fibrillary astrocyt.	90%	improved	6mo
26M	BG	Low grade astrocyt.	80%	improved	6mo
40M	BG	Glioblastoma	50%	death	
38M	F	Cavernous angioma	100%	normal	2yr
26F	P	Oligoastrocyt.	100%	improved	2yr–2P.
62M	O	Metastatic	100%	improved	1yr
33M	BG	Glioblastoma	50%	death	
43F	DF	Ganglioglioma	100%	improved	1yr
31M	DP	Glioblastoma	90%	death	
53M	F	Glioblastoma	90%	improved	6mo
9M	F	Oligodendroglioma	90%	normal	2mo
40M	F	Low grade astrocyt.	100%	improved	1mo
26M	P	Oligoastrocyt.	90%	improved	2yr
68M	O	Metastatic	100%	normal	1mo

D = deep; F, P, T, O, = convexity; BG = basal ganglia; IIIv. = third ventricle, i.v. = intraventricular; 2P = two procedures

management of these very different imaging modalities has been found to be potentially very helpful; high definition provided by MRI and CT data improves the interpretation of echographic images, now acquired along stereotactically defined planes. Shift, swelling and distortion of cerebral parenchyma, together with orientation and amount of residual tumour can be monitored intraoperatively, with successive echographic acquisitions.

Results and Discussion

The analysis of our clinical material, presented in Table 1, allows us to draw these preliminary conclusions.

Histological diagnosis, obtained with tissue biopsy, is mandatory before attempting the guided removal of a deep seated lesion; we found that poor results are mainly related to the infiltrative nature of the lesion, rather than to its anatomical location. To believe in the total removal of a malignant gliomas by following its neuroradiological contours is obviously naïve, but can also be dangerous when carried out through a narrow path that reaches down to the deep midline, where swelling of residual tumour causes devastating effects.

Low-grade gliomas and lesions with well-defined borders can be safely removed with surprisingly little postoperative morbidity, but the number of cases, in our series, in which postoperative CT revealed unexpected incomplete removal, has prompted us to search for intraoperative monitoring instrumentation.

We have found that intraoperative shift of the target due to swelling and to surgical manouvers happens more frequently to lesions in the deep convexity, than to those lying close to the midline. Intraoperative control has remarkably improved with the introduction of stereotactic echographic images.

Conclusions

The field of stereotactically guided microsurgery is definitely bound to grow in interest and increase in application. Our preliminary experience suggests that research efforts should be directed towards the development of a system which minimizes the burden of ancillary manouvers related to preoperative image acquisition, and relieves the surgeon of the demanding task of "setting angles and depths" on traditional stereotactic instruments. Furthermore, the need for intraoperative monitoring devices is strongly felt and the development of stereotactic intraoperative echographic acquisition represents a solution which can be relatively easily integrated with other preoperative stereotactic images.

References

1. Apuzzo MLJ, Sabshin JK (1983) Computer tomographic guidance stereotaxis in the management of intracranial mass lesions. Neurosurgery 12: 277–284
2. Giorgi C, Casolino D, *et al* (1981) Computer assisted planning of stereotactic neurosurgical procedures. Child's Nerv Syst 5: 299–302
3. Kelly PJ, Alker GJ (1981) Stereotactic approach to deep seated central nervous system neoplasms using carbon dioxide laser. Surg Neurol 15: 331–334
4. Reinhardt HF, Landolt H (1989) CT guided "real time" stereotaxy. Acta Neurochir (Wien) [Suppl] 46: 107–108
5. Riechert T (1980) Stereotactic brain operations: Methods, clinical aspects, indications 89: 117
6. Sedan R, Peragut JC, *et al* (1988) Guidage stereotaxique de certaines interventions a crane ouvert. Neurochirurgie 34: 97–101
7. Watanabe E, Watanabe T, *et al* (1987) Three dimensional digitizer (neuronavigator): New equipment for CT guided stereotaxic surgery. Surg Neurol 27: 543–547

Correspondence: C. Giorgi, Departments of Neurosurgery and Child Neurology, Istituto Neurologico "C. Besta", 11, Via Celoria, I-20133 Milano, Italy.

Acta Neurochirurgica, Suppl. 52, 22–25 (1991)

Trans-Fissural or Trans-Sulcal Approach Versus Combined Stereotactic-Microsurgical Approach

R. Garcia Sola, P. Pulido, and **E. Kusak**

Department of Neurosurgery, Hospital de la Princesa, Autonomous University, Madrid, Spain

Summary

The combined stereotactic-microsurgical approach has been used mainly to allow the removal of small subcortical lesions, determining their location and the route to be followed. In our experience, this approach has been most useful in 5 cases of small paraventricular AVMs and another 6 small deep-seated tumoural lesions.

Since the availability of MRI, we have systematically applied Yasargil's proposal to perform dissection of the cisterns or sulci to reach a lesion with minimal or no injury to normal neuroanatomy. Assisted by Computer Aided Design software, we can superimpose the MR images with those provided by conventional or digital angiography (mainly the venous phase). MRI allows us to select a route or pathway through a sulcus, and angiography helps us in locating it on the brain surface.

We have applied this technique systematically during the past year, and can report 20 cases (1 AVM, 12 tumoural lesions, 1 abscess and 6 haematomas). This trans-fissural or trans-sulcal approach has allowed us resection with minimal surgical damage, after a prompt and precise location.

We think that both methods are not mutually exclusive, although the trans-sulcal approach is more adequate because of less discomfort for the patient, the smaller cerebral parenchyma injury and greater anatomofunctional information for the surgeon.

Keywords: Stereotactic neurosurgery; stereotactic approach; trans-sulcal approach.

Introduction

Based on the idea suggested by Guiot[1] and further developed by Riecher[3], in 1980 we presented the case of a 42 year old patient in whom a small paraventricular arteriovenous malformation (AVM) was resected, through a combined approach (stereotactic-microsurgical)[2].

Recently, Yasargil[4] proposed the dissection of the cortical sulci and their use as an approach to deep-seated lesions. Magnetic Resonance Imaging (MRI) and the Computer Aided Design (CAD) of drawings and graphics (AUTOCAD v.9 - Autodesk Inc) allowed us to get greater confidence in the use of the trans-sulcal approach.

We report our experience with both types of approach and state their advantages and disadvantages.

Material and Method

Group A – Combined Approach (Stereotactic-Microsurgical)

The method consists basically, depending on the stereotactic frame, in the performance of angiography (in cases of AVM) or a CT scan (in tumours) under stereotactic conditions. After locating the lesion, the entrance point is chosen and a small trephine is performed. To avoid displacement of the cerebral mass, a cannula is introduced close to the lesion before the duramater is incised. Then, with a microsurgical technique, the duramater is opened and the course of the cannula which has spaced marks at 1 cm. is followed to the lesion that is then resected[2].

When using Leksell's frame, it is sometimes necessary to make a burr hole, introduce the cannula, fix it to the duramater, suture the skin, remove the frame and perform a craniotomy around the burr hole. Later, the cannula's course is followed as above. This disadvantage is solved with the newly designed Leksell's frame that permits free access to the cranial vault.

Using this method we have totally resected 4 small paraventricular AVMs using the Talairach's frame, and another small and deep-seated AVM and 6 subcortical tumours (1 astrocytoma and 5 metastases) with the Leksell's frame.

Group B – Trans-Sulcal Approach

The following methodology has been used for the access and resection of deep subcortical lesions:

1. MRI, especially the sagital views, from the midline to the outmost cortex (Fig. 1).
2. Conventional or digital angiography (without subtraction of the cranial outline), especially in the venous phase.
3. Plain x-ray films in lateral projection and CT scan, if necessary to give more information of the lesions characteristics.

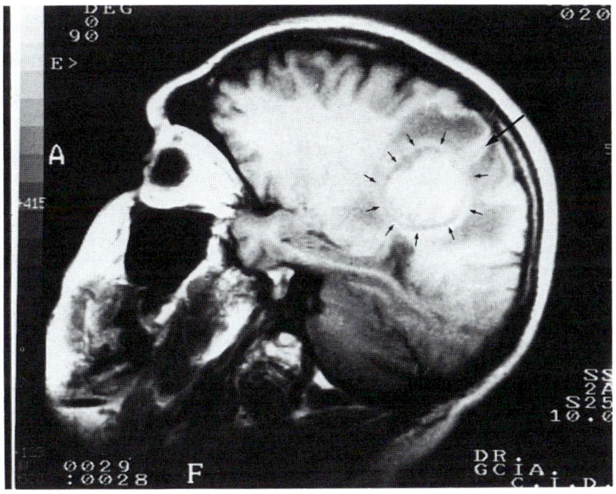

Fig. 1. Sagital view of a deep-seated metastatic lesion. A parietal sulcus approaches the lesion (arrow)

4. Using CAD software and a digitizer, a drawing is made with superimposed layers at the same scale (generally at the plain X-ray conventional size). It includes (Fig. 2):

A. – An outline of the cranial base and vault with the most important sutures and anatomical references.
B. – The arterial and venous phases of the angiogram with greatest detail of the selected zone.
C. – The lesion and its surgically relevant features: most enhancing zones, nodes, necrosis, etc.
D. – Cortical sulci most closely related to the lesion.
E. – Cerebral mapping according to J. Talairach's methodology, based on the AC-PC intercommisural line.

This design allows a bidimensional view of the lesion. Aided by the tridimensional view of the MRI, the selection of a cortical sulcus to approach the lesion can be made. Through the superimposition of the drawings layers the relation of such a sulcus with the cortical veins (easy to find after opening the duramater) and the functional areas of the affected zone can be found.

The operation consists of the performance of a centered craniotomy over the lesion, aided by the relation between the lesion and the external osseous references (sutures, orbital roof, external

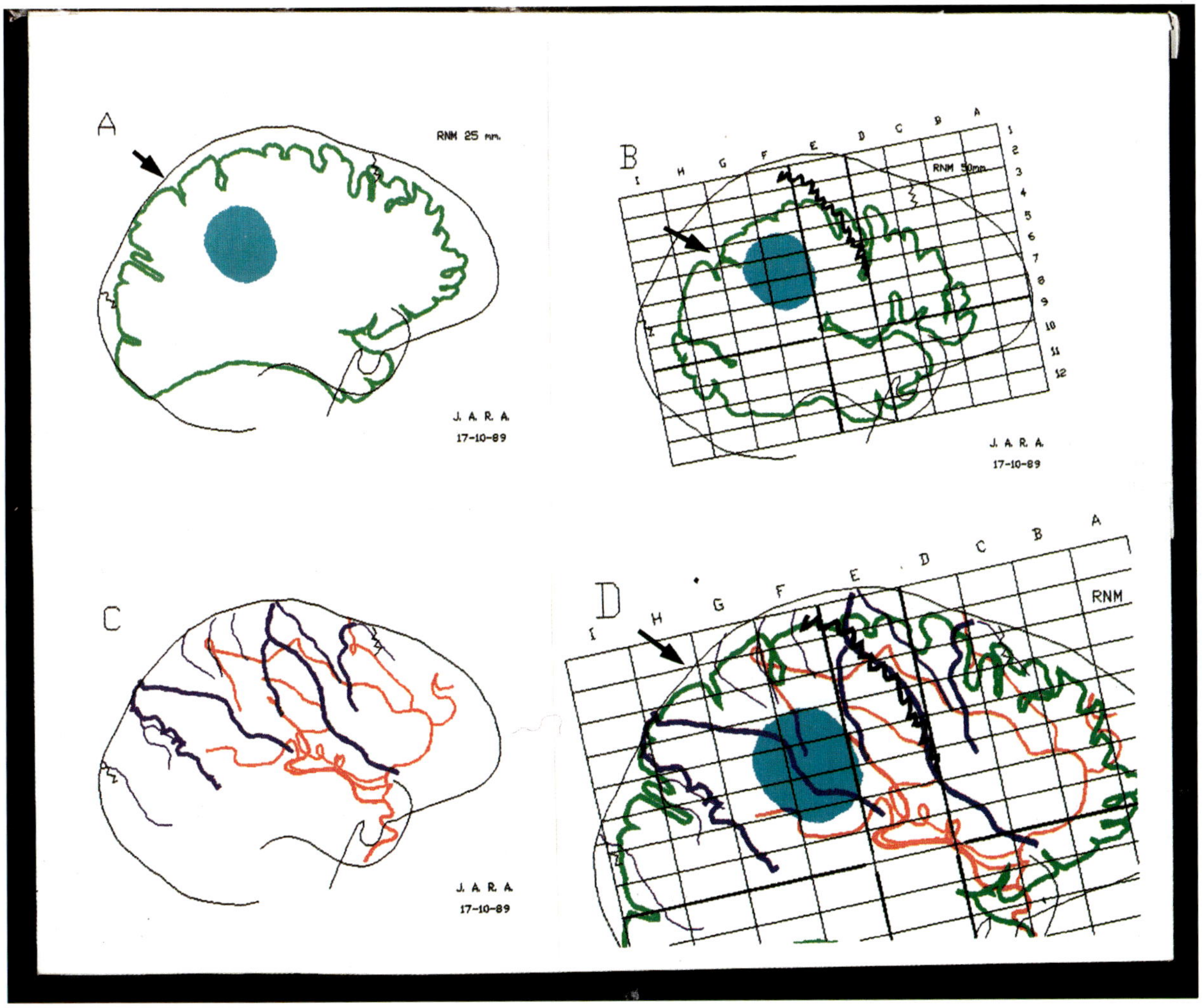

Fig. 2. CAD drawing of the same patient as in Fig. 1. A. – Plain x-ray film and sagital view of MRI at 25 mm. from midline. B. – Sagital view at 50 from midline and TALAIRACH's mapping. The selected sulcus (arrows) as approach route. C. – The arterial and venous phases of digital angiography. D. – Magnified vision of the lesion

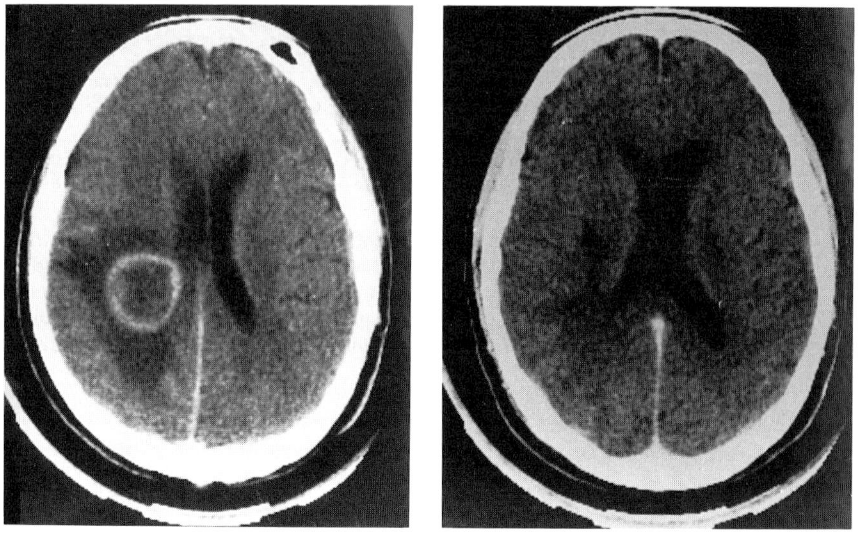

Fig. 3. Same patient as in Figs.1 and 2. Pre and postoperative CT scan

auditory canal...). After opening the duramater, the cortical veins, their configuration and the selected sulcus are located according to the drawing. The sulcus is then opened with microsurgical techniques, followed by the incision of its wall or floor depending on the lesion's location on the MRI.

In general, following the "keyhole" technique proposed by Yasargil[4], the incision should be no larger than 2 cm. Total excision is carried out with the usual microsurgical techniques, the bipolar coagulation, Co_2, Nd-YAG and contact lasers, and ultrasonic suction, depending on the macroscopic features of the lesion (Fig. 3).

In this way we have approached a small deep-seated subcortical AVM, 4 astrocytomas, 8 metastases, 1 abscess and 6 haematomas.

Results and Discussion

None of the 11 patients treated by a combined approach nor the 20 patients in whom a trans-sulcal approach was used had further neurological deficits, and all recovered from surgery within a week at most.

The lesion was found and microscopically resected in every case, confirmed with postoperative CT scans. Two cases of Group A, both very small metastatic lesions (< 2 cm.), were difficult to find, probably because the cannula moved a small distance from the lesion. In two other cases in Group B, with very small gliomas (< 2 cm.), the sulci at both sides of the gyrus where the lesion was theoretically located were opened. This allowed a greater exposure before opening the gyrus to excise the lesions.

We can summarize our impressions about the advantages and disadvantages of both methods as follows:

A – Combined Approach

I. Advantages:
- Accuracy
- Small craniotomy
- Microsurgical procedure is quick

II. Disadvantages:
- Discomfort and stress for the patient during the sterotactic calculation
- Only one radiological test in stereotactic conditions is available
- Risk of mobilization of the brain and displacement of the cannula
- Surgical field limited by the stereotactic device.

B – Trans-Sulcal Approach

I. Advantages:
- Not dependent on the Radiology Department
- All tests are superimposed and correlated
- There is no displacement of the lesion in relation with the cerebral anatomic references
- Better and more accurate anatomofunctional knowledge of the area to be operated on
- The approach is selected according to the function of the cortex
- Smaller cortical cerebral lesion.

II. Disadvantages:
- The radiological tests must be performed with the patient in the correct position
- The design and drawings are time consuming. Knowledge of the program is needed

- Less accuracy (?). It will increase with the improvement of software including real tri-dimensional possibilities
- Need for a bigger craniotomy.

In summary, we think that both methods are not mutually exclusive, although we feel the trans-sulcal approach to be more adequate because of less discomfort for the patient, the smaller lesion on the cerebral parenchyma and greater anatomofunctional information for the surgeon.

Acknowledgements

The authors wish to express their thanks to the Fundacion Ramon Areces.

References

1. Guiot G, Rougerie J, Sachs M, *et al* (1960) Repérage stéréotaxique de malformations vasculaires profondes intracérébrales. Sem Hôp Paris 36: 1134–1143
2. Garcia Sola R, Cabezudo J, Areitio E, Bravo G (1980) Combined approach (stereotactic-microsurgical) to a paraventricular arteriovenous malformation. Acta Neurochir (Wien) [Suppl] 30: 413–416
3. Riecher T, Mundinger F (1964) Combined stereotactic operation for treatment of deep-seated angiomas and aneurysms. J Neurosurg 21: 358–363
4. Yasargil M G, Cravens G F, Roth P (1988) Surgical approaches to "inaccessible" brain tumours. Clin Neurosurg 34: 42–110

Correspondence: R. Garcia-Sola, Department of Neurosurgery, Hospital de la Princesa, Autonomous University, Madrid, Spain.

Acta Neurochirurgica, Suppl. 52, 26–29 (1991)

Computer Assisted Volumetric Stereotactic Resection of Superficial and Deep Seated Intra-Axial Brain Mass Lesions

P.J. Kelly

Department of Neurosurgery, Mayo Clinic, Rochester, MN, USA

Summary

The integrated computer-based stereotactic system for volumetric resection of brain mass lesions, which has been developed by the author, is described.

The results of a series of 451 cases are presented. Morbidity was 7.7% and mortality 1%

Keywords: Brain tumour; volumetric stereotactic resection; computer assisted; results.

The advent of computer based imaging technologies brought about new options for the stereotactic diagnosis and treatment of intracranial mass lesions. Points within CT and/or MRI defined intracranial lesions can be targeted for diagnostic biopsy. In addition tumour resection can be guided by stereotactic techniques. Over the past 10 years we have developed systems and procedures for stereotactic tumour resection. In 1979 we began using stereotactic point in space localization to guide the stereotactic exposure of deep seated lesions[3,4]. However, computer reconstruction of the boundaries of a lesion detected on stereotactic CT and MRI examinations allows the representation of a lesional volume in stereotactic space. We therefore developed an integrated computer-based stereotactic system for volumetric resection of subcortical lesions[1,5,6,7]. The following describes our system and methods for stereotactic volumetric resection of subcortical lesions and the clinical results achieved over the past six year period.

Methods

Volume in Space

Patients undergo stereotactic CT, MRI and digital angiographic (DA) examinations with their heads fixed in a CT/MRI compatible stereotactic headframe. Localization systems for DA/CT/MRI create reference marks from which stereotactic coordinates for any pixel on individual images may be calculated.

The computer generated CT, MRI and DA data is transferred to the operating room computer system (SUN 4 workstation with Data General 9800 back-up and VICOM image processor). By means of a user friendly menu based program and mouse subsystem the surgeon simply traces around the contours of the tumour on serial CT slices and MR images. The computer then suspends these slices within a three dimensional image matrix which corresponds directly to the stereotactic coordinate system of the stereotactic head frame which will be used for the actual surgery. An interpolation program creates a volume for the CT and MRI defined limits of the lesion.

This volume can be sliced perpendicular to the intended surgical viewline in order to present to the surgeon the appearance of the lesion as it will be encountered at surgery. Alternatively it can be represented by a shaded graphics algorithm, rotating in space to provide the surgeon with a conceptualization of the lesion as a three dimensional volume. The lesional volume scaled to the proper image size can also be displayed in the correct location within the stereoscopic angiogram or upon a map of the brain sulci and fissures derived from the stereoscopic angiogram. Finally all of this data can be displayed within a shaded graphics rendition of the patient's skull which has been extracted from the stereotactic CT scan. Such displays are used in surgical simulations: planning the stereotactic trajectory to an intracranial lesion in order to approach and extract a tumour in the safest possible manner.

Surgical Procedures: Computer-Assisted Stereotactic Volumetric Resection

Intracranial tumours represented as CT and/or MRI defined volumes in stereotactic space can be removed with appropriate instrumentation utilizing a computer interactive method. These procedures employ a *COMPASS*™ arc-quadrant* stereotactic frame, a heads-up video display terminal attached to the operating microscope, a carbon dioxide laser system and various custom microsurgical instruments which have been designed specifically for these procedures.

* Stereotactic Medical Systems, Seneca Turnpike, New Hartford, New York.

Computer generated images of the imaging defined tumour volume sliced perpendicular to the surgical approach trajectory are projected into a head-up display unit mounted on the operating microscope. These images are scaled to the exact size of the surgical field viewed through the operating microscope and are superimposed up it. Thus, during these procedures, the surgeon views not only the surgical field itself but also a computer generated rendition of what that surgical field should look like based on the CT, MRI and DA data bases.

Computer assisted stereotactic resections can be performed in superficial and deep-seated lesions. In superficial lesions a circular trephine is turned on a stereotactically placed cranial pilot hole centered over the lesion. The trephine defect having a known configuration and size serves as a reference structure for indexing of the scaled image within the heads-up display of the operating microscope (Fig. 1). The computer generated image of the trephine with respect to the CT/MRI defined tumour volume is superimposed over the actual trephine in the surgical field viewed through the operating microscope. Thus the computer generated tumour slice images serve as a template which guides the dissection around subcortical lesions and facilitates identification of the plane between the lesion and the surrounding brain parenchyma.

Deep-seated lesions are resected by means of a stereotactically directed cylindrical retractor inserted through a dilated cortical and subcortical white matter incision. The heads-up display unit on the operating microscope is superimposed on the computer-generated slice images over the surgical field (Fig. 2). In practice a plane is developed between tumour and surrounding brain tissue before the lesion is vaporized with a high power defocused carbon dioxide laser. Lesions which are much larger than the retractor can be removed by multiple image translations on the display screen which results in the calculation of new stereotactic coordinates. These, once executed on the *COMPASS*™ stereotactic slide system, position a new part of the tumour under the stereotactic retractor.

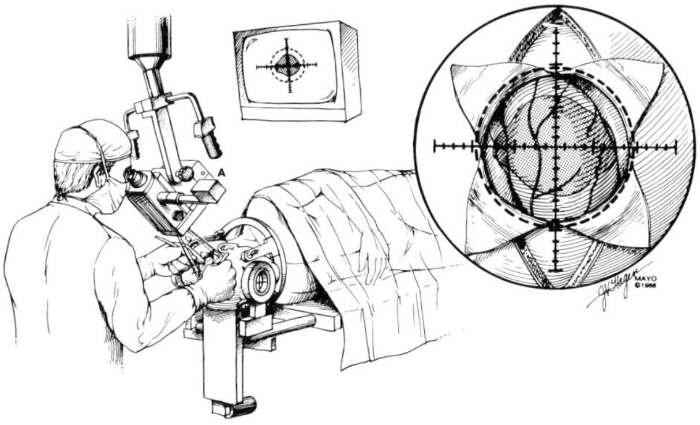

Fig. 2. Stereotactic resection of deep tumour through stereotactically directed cylindrical retractor. Computer displays on monitor and into heads-up display unit (A) tumour slices with respect to outline of retractor. (Reprinted with permission from Kelly PJ (1988) Volumetric stereotactic surgical resection of intra-axial brain mass lesions. Mayo Clinic Proc 63: 1186–1198)

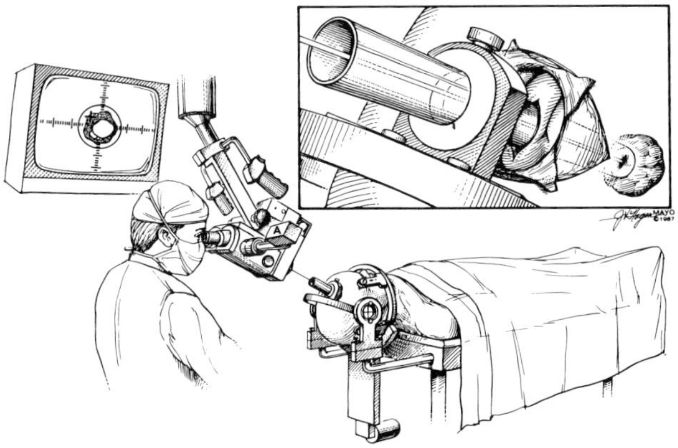

Fig. 1. Method for stereotactic volumetric resection of superficial lesions. Computer displays reformatted CT/MRI defined tumour outlines with respect to location and configuration of stereotactically placed trephine. (Reprinted with permission from Kelly PJ (1988) Volumetric stereotactic surgical resection of intra-axial brain mass lesions. Mayo Clinic Proc 63: 1186–1198)

Patient Selection

Between August 1984 and August 1990, computer assisted volumetric stereotactic resection procedures have been performed on 451 patients at the Mayo Clinic. These include 261 patients with astrocytomas (Grade IV: 84 patients, Grade III: 17 patients, Grade II: 19 patients, Grade I: 6 patients and pilocytic astrocytomas: 51 patients), 21 with mixed gliomas, 42 with oligodenrogliomas, 71 patients with metastatic tumours, 16 with meningiomas, 21 with colloid cysts, 44 with vascular lesions and a variety of miscellaneous lesions. Tumour locations are illustrated in Fig. 3. We have found that the procedure can remove any selected intracranial lesion or preselected portion thereof as assessed by postoperative CT scanning.

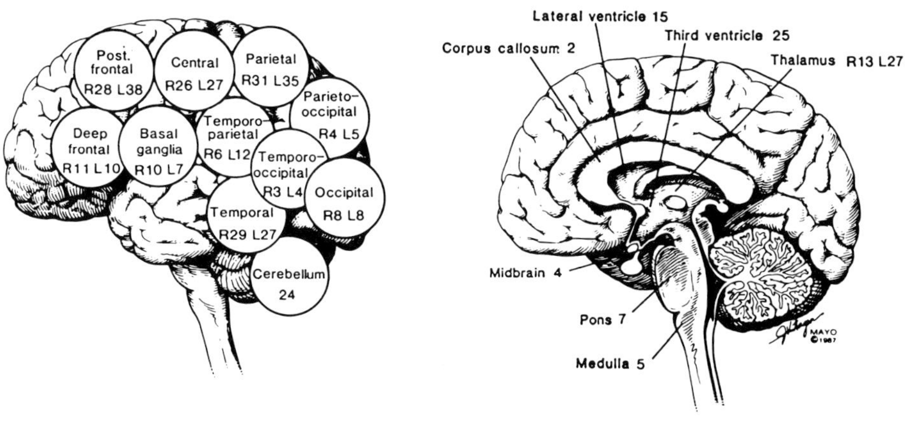

Fig. 3. Tumour locations in 451 patients undergoings volumetric stereotactic tumour resection

Results

Postoperative neurological examinations have revealed that 199 patients were neurologically improved from their preoperative level, 217 were neurologically unchanged (148 had been neurologically normal preoperatively, 69 had a preoperative neurological deficit which did not improve postoperatively) and 35 patients were neurologically worse (morbidity 7.7%). Three of these patients died within 30 days following surgery (mortality 1%).

Discussions

Computer assisted volumetric resection is most beneficial in benign circumscribed gliomas such as pilocytic astrocytomas and selected low grade oligodendrogliomas, subependymomas and in subcortical metastatic tumours. A complete gross total resection can be achieved in all of these cases as well as in other nonglial neoplasms and nonneoplastic mass lesions. The resection of infiltrative lesions is technically possible with the *COMPASS*™ system

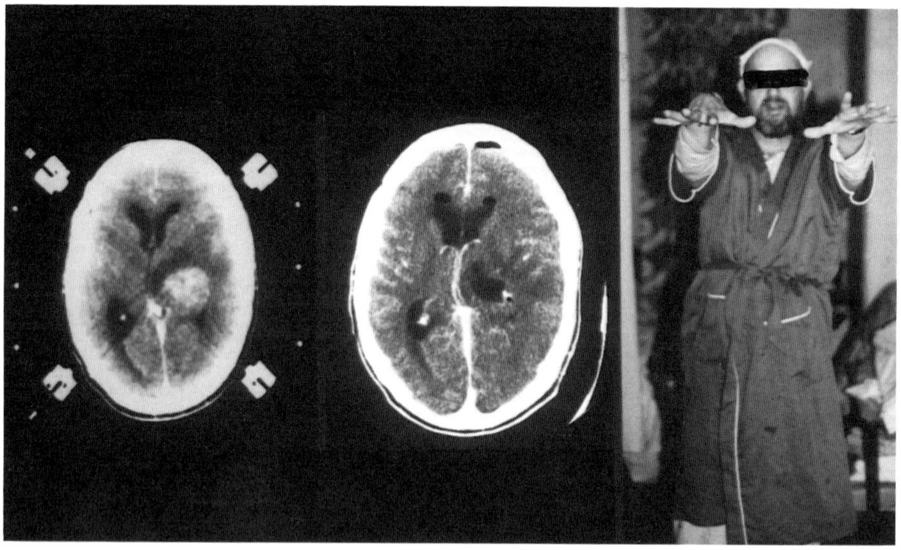

a

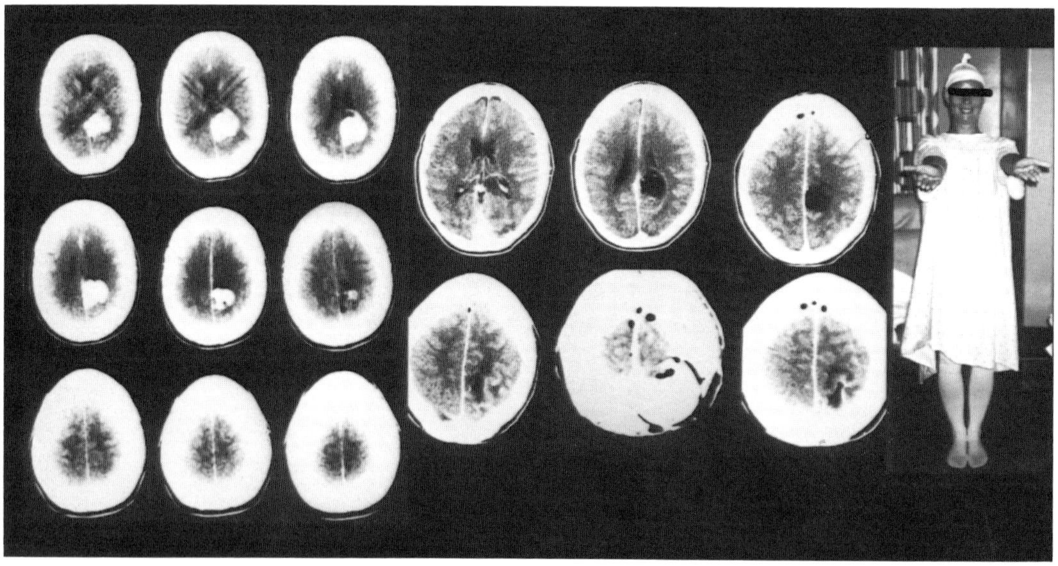

b

Fig. 4. Pre- (*left*) and postoperative (*middle*) contrast enhanced CT scans in a 43-year-old man with a left thalamic grade 4 astrocytoma (a) and a 27-year-old female with a deep left parietal pilocytic astrocytoma. (b) Both patients were photographed four days after surgery

technology. However, functional brain parenchyma infiltrated by isolated tumour cells is also resected. Thus, in important brain regions, volumetric resection is used to resect the tumour tissue components of the lesion only[2].

Volumetric stereotaxis is mathematically complex and requires interpolations, integrations, elaborate image processing and reconstructions. Even though volumetric stereotaxis can be performed utilizing inexpensive manual methods[3,4], these methods are cumbersome, time consuming and impractical on a day to day basis. With the *COMPASS*™ system, a totally integrated computer based stereotactic system, volumetric stereotactic procedures are practical, and time and cost efficient[2,5,6].

References

1. Kelly PJ (1988) Volumetric stereotactic surgical resection of intra-axial brain mass lesions. Mayo Clin Proc 63: 1186–1198
2. Kelly PJ (1990) Stereotactic imaging, surgical planning and computer assisted volumetric resection of intracranial lesions: Methods and results. In: Symon L (ed), Advances and Technical Standards in Neurosurgery, vol. 17, Springer, New York, pp 77–118
3. Kelly PJ, Alker GJ (1980) A method for stereotactic laser microsurgery in the treatment of deep seated CNS neoplasms. Appl Neurophysiol 43: 210–215
4. Kelly PJ, Alker GJ Jr (1981) A stereotactic approach to deep seated CNS neoplasms using the carbon dioxide laser. Surg Neurol 15: 331–334
5. Kelly PJ, Alker GJ Jr, Goerss S (1982) Computer assisted stereotactic laser microsurgery for the treatment of intracranial neoplasms. Neurosurgery 10: 324–331
6. Kelly PJ, Kall BA, Goerss SJ, Earnest F (1986) Computer assisted stereoxic resection of intra-axial brain neoplasms. J Neurosurg 64: 679–681
7. Kelly PJ, Goerss SJ, Kall BA (1988) Evolution of contemporary instrumentation for computer assisted stereotactic surgery. Surg Neurol 30: 204–215

Correspondence: P.J. Kelly, Department of Neurosurgery, Mayo Clinic, Rochester, MN, USA.

Acta Neurochirurgica, Suppl. 52, 30–32 (1991)

Endoscopic Procedures in Stereotactic Neurosurgery

D. Hellwig and **B.L. Bauer**

Department of Neurosurgery, Philipps-University Marburg, Germany

Summary

A new prototype of an endoscope for stereotactic interventions is described. This endoscope is adapted to the Mundinger-Birg stereotactic system. Stereotactic endoscopic procedures are carried out for brain-tumour-biopsy as well as for evacuation of haematomas, brain-cysts and abscesses. Ventriculoscopy is performed on hydrocephalus and biopsy of ventricle-relating tumours. One-year experience with stereotactic endoscopy is reviewed.

Keywords: Stereotactic neurosurgery; endoscopy; brain tumour; hydrocephalus; brain abscess.

Introduction

Endoscopy in neurosurgery is presently gaining in importance. Endoscopes are used for hematoma evacuation[1] brain tumor diagnosis and therapy[5] for interventions on hydrocephalus[2] and for aspiration of cysts[7]. Hitherto the use of endoscopic procedures in stereotaxy was limited by the large diameters of endoscopes, which is in contrast with tissue-sparing stereotactic operations.

Technical advance now makes it possible to use thin endoscopes in the practice of stereotactic neurosurgery. Since June 1989 we have performed stereotactic operations under visual control. We have reported our first results with this method elsewhere[3,4]. This is a critical evaluation of our experience with endoscopic stereotaxy after an additional year of application.

Methods

1. Instrumentation

The CT-compatible instrumentation of Mundinger and Birg is used[6]

Endoscope: The endoscopes are prototypes with diameters of 1.5 and 3.3 mm. At the moment we are using a new prototype of an ultrathin flexible endoscope, which is constructed especially for application in stereotactic neurosurgery by Olympus Inc. Tokyo. This instrument was developed in accordance with our standards which we have derived from the application of the endoscopes in stereotaxy in the the past year.

The main specifications of this instrument are: The field of view is 90°, the direction of view 0°. The Depth of field is 1–50 mm, the range of tip bending up-180° and down-100°. The insertion tube has an outer diameter of 3.3 mm. The working length of the instrument is 300 mm. There is one working channel with an inner diameter of 1.2 mm of biopsic procedures and for the application of laser-beam therapy.

Endoscope guiding-system: We have developed a special endoscope guiding-system, which is adapted to the Mundinger-Birg-System. The endoscope guide cannula is a teflon tube. This tube is transparent to give a direct view of the route of entry to the target point or region.

2. Operation-Technique

The stereotactic operation is regularly performed under local anaesthesia. The target point or region of interest is determined by computer tomography. The stereotactic operation itself is carried out in a specially equipped room. After trepanation with the stereotactically guided drill, the endoscope guide cannula with internal mandril is guided to the target point. Thereafter, x-ray pictures are made to assure proper positioning. After removing the internal mandril and introduction of the endoscope, the target region is inspected.

Visual control of the operation is possible by a connected camera.

Results

Up to now we have operated on 57 patients stereotactically under endoscopic control. The indications included: Brain tumour biopsy 33; Evacuation of haematomas 6; Drainages of cysts and abscesses 12; Ventriculoscopy 6. There have been no surgical complications, the postoperative mortality has been zero.

1. Brain Tumour Biopsy

Advantages: Stereotactic biopsies under endoscopic control are much safer.

We demonstrate that after each biopsy a small haemorrhage occurs. Most of these haemorrhages stop spontaneously, in two cases, however we had to carry out haemostatic procedures under direct view.

To avoid larger haemorrhage we inspect the target point or-region before taking a biopsy. If there is any vessel, we change the region of biopsy for some millimeters. The endoscope-guided biopsy makes it possible to discriminate normal from tumorous brain tissue. This aspect makes it easy to puncture pathological material for smear preparation diagnosis.

Disadvantages: The problem of biopsies is how clear endoscopic image can be obtained in solid brain tumour masses. We hope to solve this problem with our new endoscope which has a minimal depth of field of 1 mm.

2. Evacuation of Haemorrhages

The evacuation of haematomas under stereotactic conditions is difficult because of the small diameters of the stereotactic instruments in comparision to the generally large volume of the intracerebral bleedings.

Advantages: The use of endoscopes for stereotactic evacuations of intracerebral haematomas makes it possible to view the extent of the clot and to carry-out evacuation with rinsing and suction through the endoscope-working-channel under direct view.

We were able to evacuate nearly 50% of haemorrhages with this technique.

Intraoperative or postoperative CT-control examination, which is usually performed to observe the lytic treatment of the haematoma, is not necessary if the procedure is done endoscopically. In this way the patient is spared further extensive examinations.

Disadvantages: Clot adherence to the tip of the optical system impairs the image quality and requires constant rinsing through the working channel.

3. Drainages of Cysts and Abscesses

Advantages: The inspection of cystic cerebral processes and abscesses convey an impression of their extent. If the cyst-or abscess-material is viscous we dilute the contents and aspirate. Intraoperatively we have a visual control as to whether the cysts and abscesses are emptied. There is no more use for double-contrast cystography as it is carried out to demonstrate the complete evacuation of these processes. Furthermore we place permanent drainage-systems into cysts under endoscopic observation. If it is necessary to take biopsies of the cyst-wall or abscess-membrane for histopathological diagnosis or for microbiological investigations there is no problem in determining in the point of biopsy even if the membranes are very thin.

Disadvantages: At the moment no disadvantages are evident.

4. Ventriculoscopy

Ventriculoscopy is applied mainly for inspection of hydrocephaulus or for biopsy of ventricle-related tumours. The present aim is to get familar with the topographic relationships of the ventricular-system to find optimal approaches to different tumour localizations in the cerebral midline and to do stereotactic operations under endoscopic control in these areas with a minimal traumatization.

Laser-beam application through the working channel of the flexible endoscope is being tested now and will be of great benefit for stereotactic interventions on midline-tumours.

Conclusion

Endoscopic stereotactic procedures have been applied for a variety of neurosurgical conditions. The results are generally encouraging.

Brain tissue biopsies under visual control entail less risk of operative complications. Stereotactic haematoma evacuation with the help of endoscopy is presently being carried out. Aspiration of cysts and abscesses as well as placement of drainage-systems are appropriate indications for the application of stereotactic endoscopy. Ventriculoscopy is a meaningful contribution to operative procedures on hydrocephalus or midline tumours and it is in the process of development.

The results confirm the importance of further development in stereotactic endoscopy. This new stereotactic method is a positive addition to the classical stereotactic procedures.

References

1. Auer LM, Holzer P, Ascher PW, Heppner F (1988) Endoscopic Neurosurgery. Acta Neurochir (Wien) 90: 1–14

2. Griffith HB (1986) Endoneurosurgery-endoscopic intracranial surgery. In: Symon L, *et al* (eds) Advances and technical standards in neurosurgery Vol. 14. No 5 Springer, Wien, New York, pp 2–24
3. Hellwig D, Eggers F, Bauer BL, Likoyiannis A (1990) Endoscopic stereotaxis-preliminary results (Abstract). Stereotact Funct Neurosurg 54–55: 418
4. Hellwig D, Bauer BL, List-Hellwig E, Mennel HD Stereotactic-endoscopical procedures on processes of the cranial midline. Acta Neurochir (Wien) [Suppl] (in press)
5. Jaques S, Shelden CH, Lutes HR (1988) Computerized microstereotactic neurosurgical endoscopy under direct three-dimensional vision. In: Lunsford L D (eds) Modern Stereotactic neurosurgery. Martinus Nijhoff Publishing, Boston, pp 185–194
6. Mundinger F, Birg W (1984) Stereotactic Biopsy of intracranial processes. Acta Neurochir (Wien) [Suppl] 33: 219–224
7. Powers S K (1986) Fenestration of Intraventricular cysts using a flexible steerable endoscope and the argon laser. Neurosurgery 18(5): 637–641

Correspondence: Dr. D. Hellwig, Dept. of Neurosurgery, Philipps-University Marburg, Baldingerstraße, D-W-3550 Marburg, Federal Republic of Germany.

Transplantation

Acta Neurochirurgica, Suppl. 52, 35–38 (1991)

Towards a Neural Transplantation Therapy for Parkinson's Disease: Experimental Principles from Animal Studies

S.B. Dunnett

Department of Experimental Psychology, University of Cambridge, U.K.

Summary

Animal experimentation is necessary to identify the optimal parameters and procedures for clinical application of neural tissue transplantation. Experiments in animal models of Parkinson's disease are briefly reviewed. Embryonic nigral tissues survive transplantation well and yield good functional recovery on a variety of motor tests. The age of the donor, the implantation technique, and the site of placement in the host brain all influence graft efficacy. Nevertheless there are theoretical limits to the power of current procedures, and even under optimal circumstances full recovery cannot be expected.

Keywords: Neural transplantation; Parkinson's disease; rats; monkeys.

Introduction

Parkinson's disease involves a primary degeneration of the dopaminergic neurons of the substantia nigra. It has been known since the time of Cajal that, in the absence of neurogenesis in the adult brain, once neurons are lost (whether through trauma or degeneration) they are not replaced. Although dopaminergic drugs have been available to alleviate some of the symptoms, the course of Parkinson's disease is unremitting and the prognosis is poor. Recent animal experiments have shown that implantation of embryonic dopamine neurons can provide experimental replacement of lost neurons in animal models of parkinsonism, and functional recovery of the associated motor symptoms. There is consequently great interest in whether similar procedures may be applicable as a clinical replacement therapy for patients.

At the time of writing (August 1990) there have been at least 500 cases of adrenal autotransplantation in patients with Parkinson's disease, and another hundred or so cases receiving embryonic or foetal nigral grafts. The picture is confused, with case reports varying from great optimism to relative pessimism about the prospect of the techniques working reliably. However, perhaps the greatest difficulty in evaluating this literature is the lack of standardisation and variability in the techniques: not only in the source of donor tissue, but in the procedures for implantation, the selection of ventricular, caudate or putamen as target site for graft placement, and the methods of functional evaluation.

Many of the biological principles for optimising graft viability and efficacy have been well characterised in animal studies[15]. The "majority position" on the key principles is briefly reviewed, although in many case full concensus has not yet been reached.

Adrenal vs. Embryonic Nigra Tissues

The first studies on dopamine cell transplantation employed the developing nigral cells from embryonic donors in rats. Such grafts were found to be efficient in replacing lost dopamine neurons and providing a new dopaminergic fibre innervation of the host striatum. Dopaminergic axons growing out of the grafts made synaptic contacts with target striatal neurons; basal and stimulated levels of dopamine turnover were restored in the reinnervated striatum; and the animals recovered in behavioural tests of many of the motor symptoms induced by experimental dopamine denervating lesions.

Interest in the adrenal medulla as an alternative graft tissue arose out of the hope that it would provide an ethically less controversial source of catecholamine cells for transplantation than foetal tissue. Moreover, although the brain has been considered an immunologically privileged site, the privilege is only relative and use of adrenal autografts circumvents any histocompatibility problems that might arise.

Studies of adrenal grafts in mice, rats and monkeys all indicate that the grafts can exert a functionally beneficial effect on the host animals. However, both the viability and the efficacy of adrenal grafts is considerably less than foetal nigral grafts, and the two types of tissue probably exert their effects in somewhat different ways. In particular, adrenal grafts do not appear to work by providing dopaminergic cell replacement and reinnervation. Rather, they have been found to stimulate sprouting and regrowth of spared host dopamine fibres. As a consequences, adrenal transplantation surgery can lead to recovery of deficits even when the grafts themselves do not survive. Thus, adrenal grafts can enhance the compensatory growth of intrinsic dopamine neurons that survive the lesion, but they cannot reverse or replace the cell loss and they will not be effective in situations where denervation is extensive, as in the more advanced stages of neurodegenerative disease.

Age of Nigral Donors

Experimental studies have determined on pragmatic grounds that nigral cells survive transplantation best when taken from embryonic donors at a particular stage of development. The same stage of development is found to be optimal in different rodent and primate species (around Carnegie stages 17–21). The optimal time corresponds to the stage when the cells are undergoing final mitotic division and before they have developed extensive neurite outgrowth. It has certainly been found that tissues taken from later foetal donors can survive, especially when transplanted as solid tissue pieces rather than as dissociated cell suspensions. Nevertheless, the few studies that have explicitly compared viability across embryonic/foetal ages all demonstrate that survival from late foetal donors is poor in comparison to tissue taken from optimal embryonic stages.

Implantation Procedures

A variety of different procedures have been adopted, but fall into two main classes:

"Solid" transplants. Pieces of donor tissue are inserted as a chunk or small fragments into the depths of the brain. For this to work the graft must be placed into a richly vascularised site that can provide adequate energy and nutrients to sustain the graft tissue. The lateral ventricles provide a natural site since the space is available and the choroid plexus provides a rich blood supply. Alternatively, other sites, can be created by surgical cavitation, and these work best if the graft is implanted after a 3–6 week delay to allow a new highly-vascularised pial lining to reform over the floor and walls of the cavity.

Suspension transplants. The alternative approach is to prepare the graft tissue as a dissociated cell suspension which is injected stereotaxically. The suspension procedure has several advantages:

- Grafts can be accurately placed into deep as well as superficial striatal sites at will.
- The implantation procedure involves minimal trauma.
- Suspension grafts do not depend on providing a rich vascular supply – the normal capillary network of the brain is quite sufficient.
- Multiple placements can be made in the caudate, putamen and accumbens.

Although there are experimental manipulations that favour use of solid grafts, such as the placement of recording electrodes or injection cannulae into the grafts under visual guidance, suspension grafts are at least as efficient (and usually more so) in all situations involving dopamine cell replacement to promote functional recovery.

The Importance of Graft Placement

The neostriatal complex is functionally heterogeneous. In the same way that lesions in discrete striatal sectors have distinctive functional consequences, so also the location in which a nigral graft is placed will influence the pattern of functional recovery.

The issue of placement has been most extensively studied in rodents. In rats with extensive unilateral dopamine depletions, nigral grafts in the dorsal striatum (which receives heavy inputs from motor cortex) reverse the animals' motor bias in tests of spontaneous or drug-induced rotation, whereas nigral grafts in the lateral striatum (which receives heavy inputs from somatosenosry cortex) reverse the animals' contralateral neglect. Whereas the selection and initiation of different classes of directed responses is influenced by the various neostriatal sites, general locomotor activity is most sensitive to graft placements in the nucleus accumbens. Thus, in an animal with a wide range of symptoms associated with extensive forebrain dopamine depletion, distinct classes of symptoms are affected by grafts placed into discrete target sites. Moreover, multiple grafts have an additive effect, reversing the full range of impairments associated with each of the individual placements.

Whereas the caudate and putamen are not differentiated in rats, these nuclei are quite distinct in primate species, including man. Although transplantation studies are only just commencing in primates, a similar pattern of results to that observed in rats is now beginning to be described also in these species. Thus, preliminary data from our laboratory suggest that nigra graft placements in the caudate appear to be associated with improving the initiation and selection of unbiased movements, whereas putamen placements are more associated with the speed and timing of directed movements. Not surprisingly, multiple placements of nigral grafts into caudate, putamen and accumbens provide more extensive recovery than does placement in just one site.

Thus, the rodent and primate studies are in full accord. In any general therapeutic strategy, it will be necessary to make multiple implants to achieve a broad profile of recovery, with the possibility of selecting placements to suit the particular profile of impairment in each individual subject or patient.

It has sometimes been argued (in clinical and primate studies) that ventricular graft placement is necessary for functional efficacy. This conclusion almost certainly arises from use of poor implantation techniques, and is invalidated by the good recovery induced by suspension grafts in deep striatal sites, in both primates and rodents.

Limits of Recovery

Although complete recovery has been achieved following nigral transplantation on some behavioural tests, and substantial recovery in many other tests, there remain some situations in which it has not proved possible to achieve any recovery at all. The two main classes of test which have been resistant to recovery are (i) eating and drinking deficits induced by bilateral nigrostriatal lesions, and (ii) use of the contralateral paw in skilled independent reaching movements. The failure of recovery in these two classes of test is not obviously due either to an insufficient total dopamine replacement, or to a failure to reinnervate some critical target site. Rather, the bulk of evidence suggests that the failure is due to an incomplete restoration of nigrostriatal circuitry.

To be functionally effective, nigral grafts are placed in or near the neostriatum. In this ectopic site, the grafts provide a dopaminergic reinnervation of the denervated target, and restore function on tests that are sensitive to tonic dopaminergic activation, such as rotation bias, locomotor activiation or lateralised attention. However, in this site the grafts do not replace nigrostriatal connectivity and cannot restore patterned activity that would normally reach the neostriatum by that route. The most plausible interpretation of failures of recovery is that these tests are dependent upon patterned nigrostriatal inputs, which is supported by a variety of *in vivo* recording data.

Thus, whereas nigral grafts implanted in the neostriatum can restore many of the symptoms associated with forebrain dopamine depletion, not all functional deficits are amenable to develop bridge grafts that enable a nigral graft implanted in the host nigra to reinnervate distant striatal targets, these surgical techniques are not developed to a sufficient level of reliability to be routinely applicable in the large primate brain. It is therefore necessary to retain a degree of caution about the extent of recovery that may be expected in clinical trials using present ectopic transplantation techniques.

Validity of the Animal Models

Rats and monkeys do not contract Parkinson's disease, and animal models do not totally reproduce the human condition. Lesions made with 6-OHDA in rats or MPTP in primates do provide efficient means to denervate intrinsic forebrain dopamine systems. However:

i. They do not reproduce the more widespread patterns of degeneration that apply in advanced Parkinson's disease.
ii. The lesions are made in an acute operation in animals rather than developing progressively over years as in patients.
iii. Acute experimental lesions are prone to recover through a variety of compensatory biochemical changes in residual neurons spared by the lesions. Consequently, experimental studies typically use more extensive dopamine depletions than are ever observed clinically.
iv. Extensive bilateral dopamine depletions in animals induce severe regulatory as well as motor

impairments such that the animals are profoundly debilitated. Consequently, much experimental work employs unilateral lesions which induce measurable motor deficits on one side of the body but leave one dopamine system intact to sustain normal food and water intake and maintain good health. A similar degree of asymmetry is never seen clinically.

Thus, the animal models differ substantially from the human disease. Animal studies provide clear information on the capacity of dopamine grafts to repair dopamine denervation. However, the relevance of these studies to Parkinson's disease depends on the extent to which the human disease is indeed a primary dopamine-denervation syndrome.

References

1. Azmitia EC, Björklund A (eds) (1987) Cell and tissue transplantation into the adult brain. Ann N Y Acad Sci, Vol 495:
2. Björklund A, Stenevi U (eds) (1985) Neural grafting in the Mammalian CNS. Fernström Foundation Series, Vol 5, Elsevier, Amsterdam
3. Dunnett SB, Richards SJ (eds) (1900) Neural transplantation: from molecular basis to clinical application. Progress in Brain Research, Vol 82, Elsevier, Amsterdam
4. Gash DM, Sladek JR (eds) (1988) Transplantation into the Mammalian CNS. Progress in Brain Research, Vol 78, Elsevier, Amsterdam
5. Lindvall O (ed) Intracerebral transplantation in movement disorders. Fernström Foundation Series, Vol 17, Elsevier, Amsterdam

Correspondence: S.B. Dunnett, Department of Experimental Psychology, University of Cambridge, Downing Street, Çambridge CB2 3EB, U.K.

Acta Neurochirurgica, Suppl. 52, 39–41 (1991)

Study of the Analgesic Effects of the Implant of Adrenal Medullary into the Subarachnoid Space in Rats*

J.I. Ruz-Franzi and **J.M. González-Darder**

Department of Neurosurgery, Faculty of Medicine, University of Cádiz, Cádiz, Spain

Summary

The present study examined the effects of an implant of the adrenal medullar into the lumbar subarachnoid space in rat models of pain. The left adrenal medullar was grafted and sham animals were implanted with a piece of muscle. The experimental models of pain were electrical stimulation of the tail, paw pinch in arthritic rats, sciatic nerve transection and cervical posterior rhizotomy. Our results suggest that adrenal medullary implant reduces the pain sensitivity during the first weeks after surgery.

Keywords: Animal models; pain; adrenal medullary implant.

Introduction

In a series of experiments Sagen *et al.*[2–3] studied the analgesic effects of transplant of medullar adrenal chromaffin cells in areas of the central nervous system related with pain modulation. Ginzburg and Seltzer[1] tested the transplant of adrenal medullary into the spinal subarachoid space in a model of deafferentation pain. Vaquero *et al.*[4], described a disappointing outcome in two patients suffering from cancer pain using this surgical technique.

The aim of this experimental study was to evaluate if the autotransplant of the adrenal medullary is able to change the pain sensitivity in acute nociceptive and chronic nociceptive and deafferentation pain models.

Material and Methods

Male Wistar rats weighing 225–250 g at the beginning of the experiment were used. The study was conducted following the guidelines of the Ethics Committee of the International Association for the Study of Pain. In all animals a microsurgical lumbar laminectomy was carried out and a small slit was opened in the dorsal aspect of the duramater. Then, the left adrenal gland was carefully removed. In implanted animals, the adrenal gland was quickly placed in a vessel filled with oxygenized Ringer lactate solution where under magnification the medullar was dissected. Finally, the adrenal medullary was placed into the subarachnoid space and slid among the cauda equina roots. In sham implanted animals a small piece of muscle was used instead. The following experimental models of pain were used in the experiments: electrical stimulation of the tail, measuring three thresholds (tail-flick response, vocalization and vocalization maintained after discharge); arthritic rats where the paw pinch test was performed; section of the sciatic nerve and cervical posterior rhizotomy studying the autotomy behaviour (day of onset and mean autotomy score). The follow-up period was 28 days. At the end of the study animals were sacrified and the spine containing the implants was removed and processed for routine pathological study.

Results

Electrical Stimulation: There was a significant increase ($p < 0.01$; Mann Whitney test) in tail flick threshold 3 days after surgery (Fig. 1). Results were similar in both vocalization thresholds, increasing the threshold significantly on day 7 ($p < 0.05$; Mann Whitney test).

Paw Pinch in Arthritic Rats: Results are despicted in Fig. 2. There were no statistical differences between groups.

Sciatic Section: After sciatic section the mean day of onset of autotomy behaviour in sham animals was 2.6 ± 0.7 days and in implanted animals of 6.8 ± 3.9 days ($p < 0.05$; Mann Whitney test). The weekly average autotomy score is shown in Fig. 3(a).

Posterior Cervical Rhizotomy: The mean day of onset of autotomy was 3.7 ± 2.9 days in sham

*The work was supported by a grant of the 'Consejeria de Educación de la Junta de Andalucia'.

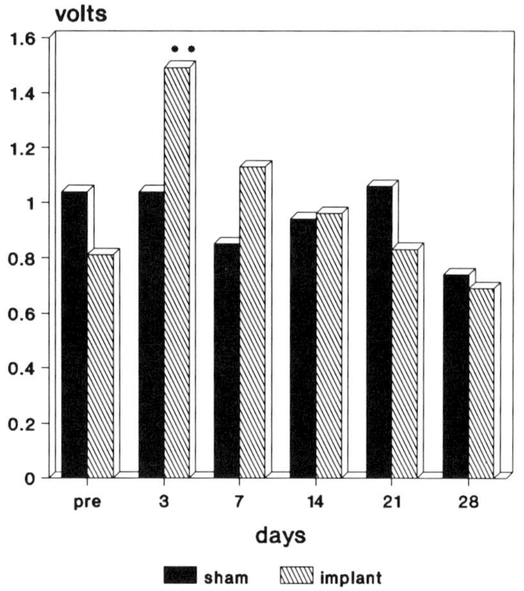

Fig. 1. Tail flick response threshold in the test of electrical stimulation of the tail in sham and implanted animals (** $p < 0.01$)

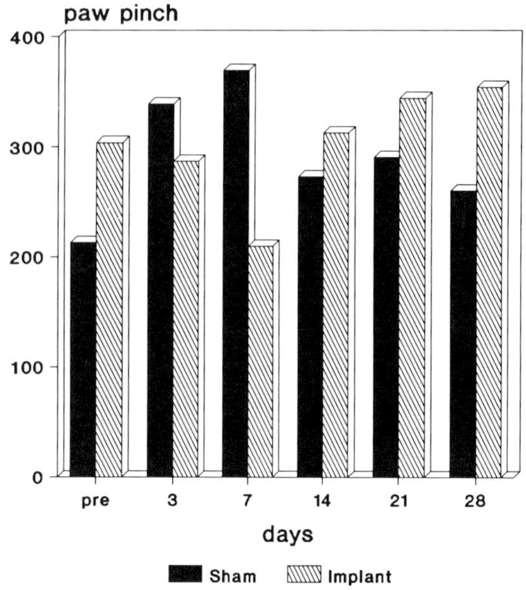

Fig. 2. Paw pinch test results in sham and adrenal medullary implanted arthritic rats

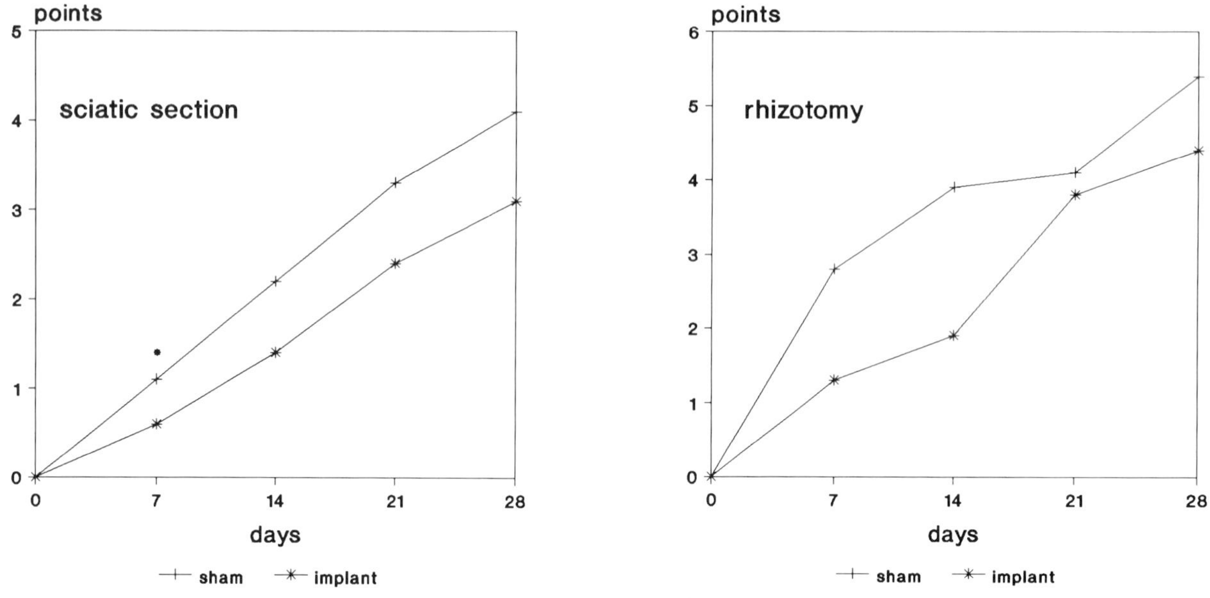

Fig. 3. Average autotomy score in sciatic sectioned (a) and cervical posterior rhizotomized rats (b). (* $p < 0.05$)

implanted animals and 6.0 ± 3.7 days in implanted rats ($p < 0.05$; Mann Whitney test). Figure 3(b) shows the mean autotomy scores reached by both experimental groups.

Pathological Study: Pathological study showed clusters of medullary cells grouped in the subarachnoid space among the roots of the cauda equina or attached in the inner aspect of the duramater.

Discussion

Our experiments on pain threshold in the test of electrical stimulation of the tail reveal no changes in pain sensitivity, excepting during the first week after surgery. On deafferentation pain models we also found changes during the first days after surgery. This would suggest some kind of transient effect of the implant modulating the pain sensitivity during the first weeks after surgery. These results are different to those described by Sagen *et al.*[2-3] and Ginzburg and Seltzer[1]. In the transplant of adrenal medulla for pain there are unfortunately few and confusing data. Obviously these contradictory results need further studies. However, transplant of the adrenal medulla into the spinal subarachnoid space and its effect on pain deserves further study.

References

1. Ginzburg R, Seltzer Z (1990) Allografting adrenal medullar of adult rats into the lumbar subarachnoid space supresses autotomy: a model of deafferentation-induced pain. Pain [Suppl 5] pp 462
2. Sagen J, Pappas GD (1987) Morphological and functional correlates of chromaffin cell transplants in CNS pain modulatory regions. In: Azmitia EC, Björklund A (eds) Cell and tissue transplantation into the adult brain. Ann N Y Acad Sci 495: 306–333
3. Sagen J, Wang H, Pappas GD (1990) Adrenal medullary implants in the rat spinal cord reduce nociception in a chronic pain model. Pain 42: 69–80
4. Vaquero J, Martínez R, Oya S, Coca S, Salazar FG, Colado MI (1989) Pain relief in humans by chromaffin tissue graft into medullary arachnoid. Transplante 1: 39–42

Correspondence: J.M. González-Darder, Department of Neurosurgery, Faculty of Medicine, E-11002-Çádiz, Spain.

Acta Neurochirurgica, Suppl. 52, 42–44 (1991)

Transplantation of Cultured Fetal Adrenal Medullary Tissue into the Brain of Parkinsonian

R. Ben, F. Ji-Chang, B. Yao-Dong, L. Yie-Jian, and **Z. Yi-Fang**

Department of Neurosurgery and Endocrinology, Dalian Municipal Central Hospital, Dalian, China

Summary

In an experimental study human fetal adrenal medullary tissue was cultured and its cytoplasmatic catecholamine storing vesicles, NA and dopamine (DA) concentration controlled for 8 days. High secretory function of DA was maintained.

This cultured human fetal tissue was transplanted to the subcortex of adult rabbits. Some of the crafts survived several months and maintained secretory function.

In a clinical study 17 patients with Parkinson's disease received a transplantation of human fetal adrenal medullary tissue, which was cultured for one week and then transplanted into the head of both caudate nuclei. During follow-up of 3–18 months all of them improved.

Keywords: Parkinson's disease; human fetal adrenal medullary tissue; transplantation.

The most characteristic pathological changes in Parkinson's Disease (PD) are neural cell loss in the substantia nigra and locus ceruleus. Associated with this morphological alteration are a number of biochemical abnormalities; the reduction in dopamine (DA) and its metabolites in the caudate nucleus. The disease is manifest by four major signs, tremor, cogwheel rigidity, akinesia, and loss of postural or balance reflexes. L-Dopa administration is the most favourable and effective treatment of PD in the last twenty years. However, when L-Dopa treatment is extended over long periods such as five to seven years, unfavourable dyskinesia or severe gastrointestinal side effects often appear. In recent years, brain transplantation of DA secreting cells has become one of the promising methods for repairing disturbance in DA metabolism both in basic neuroscience research as well as in clinical practice.

In a previous paper, the sequelae of the transplantation of the autologous adrenal medulla and the fetal substantia nigra to the caudate nucleus or to the putamen have been described. PD occurs predominantly in older patients and it is difficult to advise two major simultaneous operations i.e. a laparotomy and a craniotomy and the adrenal medulla in older patient trends to senile degeneration. The volume and the purity of grafting autologous tissue and the fetal mesencephalon tissue are not perfect in practice. Transplanting the cultured fetal adrenal medullary tissue could be an alternative way, particularly because such transplantation has been quite successful in various animal models, considerably reducing surgical risk and provides tissue with sufficient volume and purity for graft.

We report the results of grafting human fetal adrenal medullary tissue cultured to the subcortex of adult rabbits and to the head of caudate nucleus in seventeen patients with PD. Approval was obtained from the local government and research committees of our hospital, and written consent from the patients and their relatives. The patients were evaluated by means of video, measurement of NA and DA concentration in CSF, immunological aspects, electroencephalogram (EEG), somatosensory and visual evoked potentials (SEP, VEP), neuropsychological testing, CT scanning and the critical analysis of the disability in PD.

Experimental Studies

Human fetal adrenal medullary tissue was removed from fetus donated or aborted at the age of 16, 20 and 24 week's gestation. The adrenal medulla was cut into 1 mm^3 fragment and cultured in RPMI 1640 medium with 10% calf serum for two weeks. The volume of adrenal medullary tissue in fetus of 16 and 20 week's gestation was 25–40% and 50–70% of that in 24 week's gestation. The cytoplasmic catecholamine storing vesicles were less in that of 16 and 20 week's gestation as seen under the electromicroscope. In contrast, the NA and DA concentration in the medium were 1.1 ng/ml and 6.5 ng/ml through 16 weeks, then increased to 2.4 ± 1.4 ng/ml and 14.3 ± 3.3 ng/ml respectively by 24 weeks. A very intense green to yellow fluorescence was given by adrenal medullary tissue by SPG method. The greatest DA concentration in the medium was 14.3 ± 3.3 ng/ml at the 8th day, and approximately equal to the secreting DA of the tissue which was 1.4 ng/mg/24h. The NA content in the medium was 60.7% of that of DA at second day and decreased to 17% by the 8th day. These results suggest that the adrenal medullary tissue cultured from the 24 weeks gestation fetus has high functional secretory of DA.

We transplanted the human fetal adrenal medullary tissue cultured from the aborted fetus donor, aged 24 weeks gestation, to the subcortex in twenty four adult rabbits. Under the specific condition of our experiment, the grafts survived in three animals, and part graft survived in one among four animals tested at the first week after operation. In six of the animals the graft survived in others and part graft survived in one, and the graft did not survived more than one month after transplantation. In five of the ten animals the graft survived and part graft survived in one, and the graft disappeared in others by three months after grafting. These grafted cells contained catecholamine storing vesicles of chromaffin cells and had the presence of specific glyoxic acid-induced catecholamine fluorescence. This is the first demonstration that the human fetal adrenal medullary tissue cultured can survive implantation into the subcortex of the adult rabbit.

Clinical Research

The patients fulfilled the following criteria, (1) they were under 75 years of age, (2) had PD with rigidity and hypokinesia as major symptoms, (3) responded to L-dopa, but with suffered side effects, (4) Brain CTs showed no evidence of local damage or ventricular enlargement.

The NA concentration in the CSF of 30 normals and 23 parkinsonians was measured by the fluorophotometry, and showed the change of DA in CSF of the 17 parkinsonians who received the transplantation 1, 3 and 6 weeks prior and after operation. The NA concentration in CSF of normal was 3.6 ± 1.5 ng/ml and DA was 13.5 ± 3.2 nl/ml. The NA of parkinsonism CSF was 1.9 + 1.1 ng/ml and DA was 3.1 + 1.4 ng/ml. The effect of variation of DA on clinical symptoms was more significant than NA. The lower the DA concentration was, the more serious the symptom was. The DA concentration increased in 14 and was unchanged in 3 patients. The mean concentration in all patients was 8.0 + 2.8 ng/ml after surgery. It was 155% higher than that preoperatively. These findings suggest that the grafted fetal tissue is survival and can secrete DA.

In serum the IgG, IgM, C_3, CH_5O, LTT, EtRe and T cell subsets in 16 parkinsonians and 7 parkinsonians undergoing the transplantation were determined before and after surgery. IgM, C_3 and CH5O in patient were found at high levels and high titers, and IgG, IgA, LTT, EtRe and T cell subsets were found at low levels and low titers. Only IgM increased one week postoperatively, but it was as high as the preoperation level three weeks postoperatively. The others were unchanged postoperatively. These data support the view that the pathogenesis of PD is immunological disorder and the brain is an immunological privileged site for transplantation.

EEG, SEP and VEP were performed in 13 parkinsonians and 5 parkinsonians who accepted the grafting. The rate of mild abnormal EEG was 54%. The rate of delay of latency in SEP was 39%, while the rate of decrement of the amplitude was 62%, 9 of 13 patients had abnormal VEP (69%). EEG, SEP and VEP which reflects the functional state of mescencephalon and basal ganglion, the derangement of neurotransmitter, and depression of brain function. EEG, SEP and VEP improved to some degree after grafting. This result suggests that the transplantation improves the neurophysiological function of basal ganglion and brain.

The neurophysiological tests show that parkinsonian suffered from the frontal lobe-type deficits on varying degree, intellectual impairment, memory disorders, and visuospatial and visuoperceptual deficience. Postoperative tests in 8 patients, carried out 1 and 3 months after neurosurgery, revealed a significant amelioration of the clinical symptoms and the frontal lobe-type deficits, as well as an improvement in intellectual function and memory. The transplantation can partially restore the neuropsychological function in parkinsonian.

The fetal adrenal medullary tissue removed from the

fetus donor aborted at the age of 24 weeks was cultured for one week. Approximately 200–300 mg tissue were placed at the head of both caudate in 17 severe patients with PD. Their mean age at the time of transplantation was 57 years (range 38–74); their mean duration of PD onset was 8 years (range 5–13), their mean Webster disability scores was 23 (range 19–30).

Follow-up study lasted 3 to 18 months. Clinical improvement was observed in all patients and the mean of total Webster disability score was 7 3 months after grafting. According to our clinical critical analysis, the clinical efficacy was significant downward and one of seventeen patients relapsed, and the response rate of transplantation was 93% in 6 months. The response rate of 6 to 12 months was 88%. No significant variation was found in the clinical efficacy from 6 to 12 months postoperatively. Immediately after operation the drugs were withheld, but in one of five patients who were receiving their postoperative Madopar 1500 mg/day compared with 750 mg/day by the end of 3 months after operation parkinsonian symptoms reappeared. Two of twelve patients who were intolerant and unresponsive to the drug developed, or were unable to continue taking the drug because of severe side effects got satisfactory response to Madopar 500–750 mg/day. The clinical improvement of the others was unchanged without receiving Madopar. The low density areas in the head of caudate nucleus was found by examination using CT within 1 to 10 and disappeared one month after operation. The grafts survive in the brain.

Conclusions

This research has demonstrated that the human fetal adrenal medullary tissue cultured is of good function and survives in the subcortext of rabbit judged by the examination of morphology and function of grafts. In the parkinsonian who accepted the grafting of the fetal adrenal medullary tissues cultured to the head of caudate nucleus, we found increase of DA concentration in CSF, unchangeableness in immunological aspects, improvement in EEG, SEP and VEP and in neuropsychological aspect on some degree after transplantation. The PD symptoms improved markedly and were stable, comparatively L-dopa was stopped or greatly reduced after surgery.

We conclude that homograft can survive in the human brain and is associated with functional effect. The transplantation to the brain tissue is a useful method on the treatment of PD.

Correspondence: R. Ben, Department of Neurosurgery and Endocrinology, Dalian Municipal Central Hospital, Dalian, China.

Acta Neurochirurgica, Suppl. 52, 45–47 (1991)

Adrenal Medulla Autograft in Caudate Nucleus as Treatment for Parkinson Disease

G. Broggi[1], **F. Pluchino**[1], **L. Gennari**[3], **S. Geminiani**[2], **F. Tamma**[2], and **T. Caraceni**[2]

Departments of [1]Neurosurgery, [2]Neurology, Istituto Neurologico "C. Besta" Department of [3]Oncological Surgery, Istituto Nazionale dei Tumori, Milano, Italy

Summary

The personal experience of four Parkinson's disease patients operated on with adrenal medulla autograft in the caudate nucleus is reported. Results on long term, possible only in two patients, are moderately fair.

Keywords: Parkinson's disease; adrenal medulla autograft; results.

Introduction

The hypothesis and the consequent studies of auto-allograft of neuronal cells into the C.N.S. took shape first in 1890[16]. Further studies indicated the possible survival of the graft and the building of reciprocal interconnections[3,9].

In the Eighties, Swedish scientists[3] proposed and executed[2–13] the adrenal mudulla autograft, with stereotactic technique, in Parkinson patients. More recently Madrazo et al. have described a relevant improvement in clinical conditions in Parkinson patients following adrenal mudulla autograft via open cranial surgery[14]. Other Authors successfully re-utilized this technique[1,7,15].

The aim of this study is to report the experience at the Istituto Neurologico "C. Besta" on 4 cases of Parkinson disease patients treated with adrenal medulla autograft via a combined stereotactic and open surgery approach.

Material and Methods

Four patients affected from Parkinson disease, all L-Dopa responders, at various stages (Table 1) have been operated on, from February 1988 to February 1989. Selection criteria have been: complicated Parkinson; age under 65 years; very good general condition; no mental deterioration; informed consent.

Presurgery Evaluation Consisted of:

- Parkinson disease assessment with CURS (Columbia University Rating Scale), UPDRS (Unified Parkinson Disease Rating Scale), NUDS (Northwestern University Disability Scale), Hoehn and Yahr staging, on-off subjective evaluation, WAIS assessment.
- Abdominal and brain CT scan; brain MRI; EEG; cardiological assessment (EKG, dynamic EKG, bidimensional echodoppler); adrenal medulla functional assessment (blood and urinary cortisol dosage, insulin tolerance test).

Surgical technique consisted of:

- Stereotactic placement of a silastic catheter to the caudate nucleus target, with the aim to make the approach to the target easier and to prepare a "pocket" for the autograft.
- Two or three days later a double surgical procedure was carried out. A left partial adrenalectomy by means of a trans-peritoneal approach was carried out by a general surgical team. At the same time a right frontal craniotomy with a transventricular approach, made easier by the catheter, to the caudate nucleus was being performed by a neurosurgical team with microsurgical technique. The adrenal medulla was carefully dissected under the microscope and 1–2 mm^3 were "implanted" into the caudate nucleus pocket, after the removal of the catheter, and fixed by a silver haemoclip.

The pharmacological regimen (L-Dopa) was reduced to the 0.33% from the 1st to the 10th postoperative day afterwards it was increased following clinical evolution. Post-operative evaluation consisted of clinical examinations after 3 weeks, 2,6,12 and 24 months. Brain CT scan was done 3 weeks after surgery and insulin tolerance test 2 months after surgery.

Results

A short term assessment has been performed on all[4] patients, but only patients 1 and 4 have been followed

Table 1. *Patients' Characteristics*

	Case 1	Case 2	Case 3	Case 4
Age	51	61	52	46
Sex	male	female	male	male
Duration of illness	12	21	10	16
Duration of treatment	3	13	10	15
Duration of motor fluctuation	1	11	4	10
Hoehn & Yahr stage	ON = II OFF = III	ON = IV OFF = V	ON = II OFF = III	ON = II OFF = V
Motor fluctuation	wearing off mobile dystonia peak-of-dose dysk. freezing	on-off peak-of-dose dysk.	on-off diphasic dyskinesia peak-of-dose dysk.	peak-of-dose dysk. diphasic dyskinesia dystonia
Therapy	Sinemet 687.5 mg/d Mantadan 200 mg/d Akineton 4 mg/d	Sinemet 812.5 mg/d	Sinemet 750 mg/d	Sinemet 1125 mg/d Parlodel 50 mg/d right thalamotomy (11 years ago)

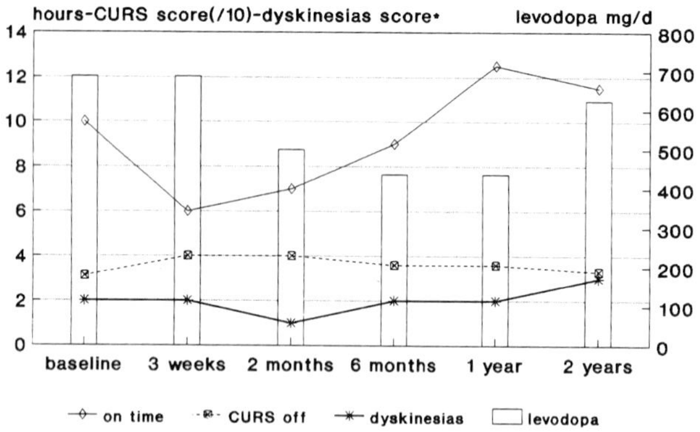

Fig. 1. Motor evaluation before and after graft Case 1

on long term range. Patient 1 had on-off fluctuation unchanged but with lower L-Dopa daily dosage. The disease, which had been rapidly progressive in the 12 preoperative months, stabilized. The patient reported and is still reporting good global improvement of his clinical conditions. His social life also improved (Fig. 1).

- Patient 4 showed progressive increase of on-periods, with unmodified dyskinesias, at the preoperative L-Dopa daily dosage.

Patients 2 and 3 did not show any particular change in their clinical status in the short term. Long term follow up is irrelevant since case 2 was lost and case 3 died 18 months after surgery from a broncopneumonia unrelated to the surgical treatment.

Postoperative assessment has been carried out with the same scales reported for the preoperative one. Surgery did not cause any mortality or morbidity, except an asyntomatic small intraparenchimal haematoma on the frontal pole in the case 1. In particular no neurological, cognitive or endocrinological side effects have been reported. A degree of analgesia and euphoria noticeable immediately after surgery disappeared in 1–2 weeks. Transient delusion appeared in the same period.

Discussion

Our data is less impressive that the ones reported by Madrazo (8) since no patient showed relevant improvement of his clinical conditions.

Nevertheless, an increase of on-off ratio at preoperative pharmacological L-Dopa dosage or an on-off ratio similar to the preoperative one, but with lower L-Dopa dosage, was observable in two patients. These results were prominent in patients 1 and 4, who also reported subjective relevant improvements which were not confirmed by the nurses and doctors assessment. No important side effects on neurological, endocrinological and psychic status were present.

Our hypothesis over these moderately fair results may be the following.

1. Necrosis of the graft, due to lack of revascularization or to anoxic damage during surgery. Actually no long term survival of the graft at the autopsy[10] or at PET scan[8] have been noticed.
2. Adrenal medulla function may be too low in Parkinson patients[6].
3. The caudate nucleus may not be the right site for

implanting the graft[12]: putamen would presumable be better[13].

4. The selection of patients may be different.

However, in conclusion, the reported experience, not completely satisfactory on the clinical side, is relevant on the surgical aspect. Better patient selection, timed allograft by means of tissue or cell bank, or fetal graft[11] should be take key to improve this fascinating approach to the neurological "degenerative" disease treatment.

References

1. Allen GS, Gurns RS, Tulipan NB, Parker RA (1989) Adrenal medullary transplantation to the caudate nucleus in Parkinson's disease. Arch Neurol 46: 487–491
2. Backlund EO, Granberg PO, Hamberger B, *et al* (1985) Transplantation of adrenal medullary tissue to striatum in Parkinsonism. First clinical trials. J Neurosurg 62: 169–173
3. Bjorklund A, Stenevi U (1979) Reconstruction of the nigrostriatal dopamine pathway by intracerebral nigral transplants. Brain Res 177: 555–560
4. Bjorklund EO, Lindvall O, Isacson O *et al* (1987) Mechanism of action of intracerebral neural implants: studies on nigral and striatal grafts to the lesioned striatum. TINS 10 (12) 509–516
5. Brundin P, Strecker RE, Lindvall O *et al* (1989) Intracerebral grafting of dopamine neurons. Ann NY Acad Sci 495: 473–495
6. Cervera P, Rascal O, Ploska A *et al* (1988) Noradrenaline, adrenaline and tyrosine hydroxylase in adrenal medulla from Parkinsonian patients. J Neurol Neurosurg Psychiatry 51: 1104–1105
7. Goetz CG, Olanow CW, Koller WC *et al* (1989) Multicenter study of autologous adrenal medullary transplantation to the corpus striatum in patients with advanced Parkinson's disease. N Engl J Med 320: 337–341
8. Guttma M Burns RS, Martin WRW *et al* (1989) PET studies of Parkinsonian patients treated with autologous adrenal implants. Can J Neurol Sci 16: 305–309
9. Halasz B, Pupp L, Uhlarik S *et al* (1963) Growth of hypophysectomized rats bearing pituitary transplant in the hypothalamus. Acta Physiol Hung 23: 287–292
10. Hirsh EC, Duykaerts C, Javoy-Agid F *et al* (1990) Does adrenal graft enhance recovery of dopaminergic neurons in Parkinson's disease? Ann Neurol 27: 676–682
11. Hitchcock ER, Kenny BG, Henderson BTH *et al* (1991) A series of experimental surgery for advanced Parkinson's disease by foetal mesencephalic transplantation. Acta Neurochir (Wien) [Suppl] 52: 54–57
12. Kish SJ, Shannak K, Hornykiewicz O (1988) Uneven pattern of dopamine loss in the striatum of patients with idiopathic Parkinson's disease. Pathophysiologic and clinical implications. N Engl J Med 318: 876–880
13. Lindvall O, Backlund EO, Farde L *et al* (1987) Transplantation in Parkinson's disease: two cases of adrenal medullary grafts to the putamen. Amm Neurol 22: 457–468
14. Madrazo I, Drucker-Colin R, Diaz V *et al* (1989) Open microsurgical autograft of adrenal medulla to the right caudate nucleus in two patients with intractable Parkinson's disease. N Engl J Med 316: 831–834
15. Motti EDF, Silani V, Scarlato G *et al* (1988) Surgical lesions, parkinsonism, and brain graft operations. Lancet ii: 346
16. Thompson WG (1890) Successful brain grafting. NY Med J 51: 701

Correspondence: G. Broggi, Department of Neurosurgery, Istituto Neurologico "C. Besta", Via Celoria, 11, 1–20133 Milano, Italy.

Acta Neurochirurgica, Suppl. 52, 48–50 (1991)

A Comparative Evaluation of Clinical Rating Scales and Quantitative Measurements in Assessment pre and post Striatal Implantation of Human Foetal Mesencephalon in Parkinson's Disease

B.T.H. Henderson, B.G. Kenny, E.R. Hitchcock, R.C. Hughes, and **C.G. Clough**

Department of Neurosurgery, University of Birmingham, Smethwick, U.K.

Summary

Six patients with advanced Parkinson's Disease were evaluated before and after implantation of human fetal ventral mesencephalic tissue to the head of the right caudate nucleus. The results of clinical assessment indicate that attempts to characterise patient fluctuations requires a combination of clinical rating scales and timing of specific limb tasks.

Keywords: Parkinson's disease; neural transplantation; clinical assessment.

Introduction

Successful intracerebral implantation of neural tissue in rodent[1,8] and non-human primate[9] models has led to clinical trials[4,5,6] in human subjects with Parkinson's disease (PD). The aim of transplantation is to develop potential therapeutic strategies; current trials have sought to establish the safety of present techniques, examine the mechanisms of clinical effects and demonstrate whether principles developed in laboratory studies can lead to a therapeutic effect in human subjects. Dopamine (DA) depletion in the striatum is the principal neurochemical deficit in PD and animal models have been designed to provide consistent host conditions for grafting experiments. In the rodent model selective unilateral striatal DA depletion and denervation has allowed reproducible pharmacological quantification of functional effects and testing of optimum donor techniques[2]. Animal models cannot reproduce the natural history, histopathology and spectrum of signs and symptomatology that occur in PD. This inherent variability makes the human subject a less consistent host for experimental transplantation surgery. The interaction of L-dopa with PD results in an increasing complexity of drug effects manifest clinically as fluctuation in motor state which is the hallmark of L-dopa treated patients[7]. Clinical assessment is critical in defining host disease patterns and in determining the character and magnitude of changes following transplantation.

Material and Methods

In 1988 twelve patients with advanced PD were assessed following stereotactic implantation of foetal ventral mesencephalon to the head of the right caudate nucleus[5]. In six of these (male/female ratio 5: 1; age range 53–67 years; mean duration of disease 18 years) inpatient clinical assessment for periods of one to six weeks prior to surgery, and at three, six and twelve months following surgery allowed comparison of two clinical rating scales and timing of specific limb tasks. All were Hoehn and Yahr grade 4 or 5 in "off" phases with different degrees of disability.

Examinations were performed on random occasions, several times daily, by the same neurologist. The duration of hospital observation enabled characterisation of individual patient fluctuations using the Webster rating scale[10] (WRS) and The North Western University Disability Scale[3] (NUDS). Asymmetry in limb rigidity, bradykinesia, and tremor were recorded as a modification of the WRS (PD score) and a further scale used to assess dyskinesia. At each examination the time to perform pronation and supination of the forearm, and to tap each foot, twenty times, was recorded.

Results

Table 1, illustrates improvement from preoperative state in all parameters in all six patients; statistical analysis was performed using the Wilcoxon signed rank pair test. Figure 1 illustrates timed limb movements and NUDS "on" scores in a patient with

Table 1. *Results*

Variable		3 months p value	6 months p value	12 months p value
NUDS "ON"		≦0.05	≦0.05	NS
NUDS "OFF"		NS	NS	NS
WRS "ON"		≦0.025	NS	NS
WRS "OFF"		NS	≦0.05	NS
Pro/Sup	Right	NS	≦0.05	≦0.025
	Left	NS	≦0.05	≦0.05
Foot tap	Right	≦0.05	NS	NS
	Left	≦0.05	NS	NS

NS = Not Statistically Significant (Wilcoxon signed rank pair test)

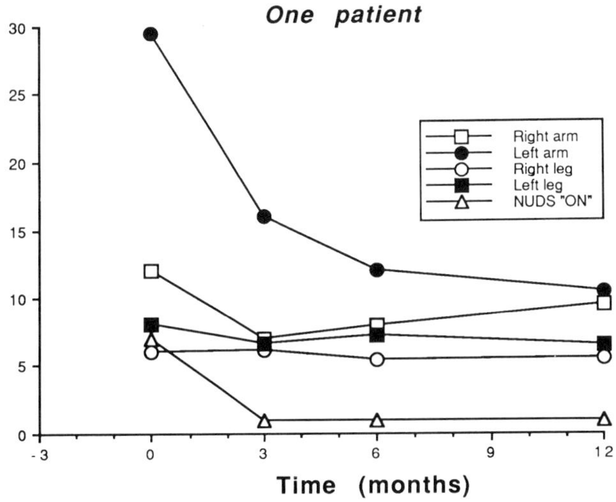

Fig. 1. Clinical Rating Scales & Timed Motor Responses

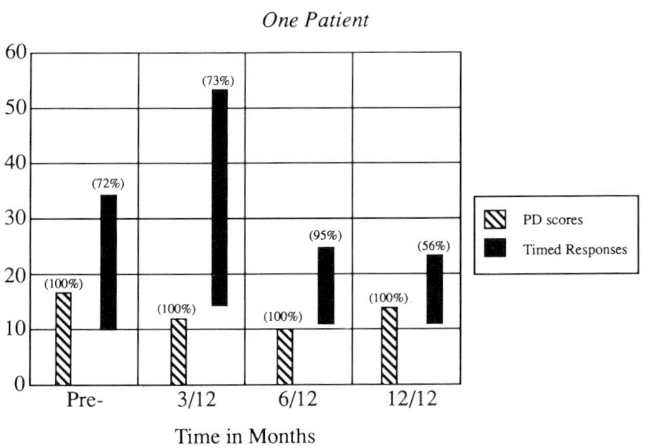

Fig. 2. High/Low Clinical Rating Scales, Timed Responses: (% Success Rate)

mild motor fluctuation and Fig. 2 the percentage success rate in performing timed motor tasks compared to PD scores in another patient with severe disability and complex fluctuation.

Discussion

Intracerebral implantation of human foetal dopaminergic tissue has potential therapeutic value in PD. With the development of consistently successful methods of collection, preparation and storage of donor material, host disease pattern will be the main influence on clinical outcome. Variability in each patient and between patients resulting from different patterns of disability and underlying disease modified by chronic L-dopa therapy is the major problem in assessment. In the patient with mild fluctuation (Fig. 1) significant improvement in contralateral timed motor limb tasks was demonstrated early and continued up to one year. There was close correlation with clinical ratings to three months but the subsequent change was not matched by improvement in disability. This lack of correlation was observed in all patients (Table 1) and was particularly apparent in those with severe disability and complex fluctuation who could only be assessed at all times by clinical rating (Fig. 2).

History taking, examination, and observation, are the main methods of obtaining clinical data but duration of "on" hours can only be calculated from patients subjective recordings. The need for repeated objective sampling over long time periods has prompted the use of quantitative measures of motor function. Such tests may have particular relevance to transplantation in PD; unlike pharmacological therapy, grafts are targeted to specific striatal sites and a lateralised effect can be differentiated. They can be recorded by paramedical staff, are sensitive and simple to perform, and are less influenced by patient and observer bias. Indices of limb function are the final common pathway of complex interactions between poorly understood cortical and subcortical pathways. Specific aspects of quality of limb movement bear little relation to patient symptoms. Clinical rating scales, although subjective, remain standard methods of assessment[3,10]. They can always be used to compare any aspect of PD in any patient although modification of scales may invalidate intergroup comparison.

Comparable and consistent assessment over the whole spectrum of disease severity is vital in quantifying the success of experimental foetal implantation in PD. We believe that this can only be accomplished by the use of both assessment methods. The mechanism of graft effects can be inferred but not proven; clinical rating scales are the most relevant method of measuring these effects.

Acknowledgements

We thank all the staff at MCNN for their assistance in the care of these patients and Mr A Rose and Mr W Mitchell for their invaluable help with illustrations.

References

1. Bjorklund A, Stenevi U (1979) Reconstruction of the nigrostriatal dopamine pathway by intracerebral nigral transplants. Brain Res 177: 555–560
2. Brundin P, Strecker RE, Widner H *et al* (1988) Human fetal dopamine neurons grafted in a rat model of Parkinson's disease: immunological aspects, spontaneous and drug-induced behaviour, and dopamine release Exp Brain Res 70: 192–208
3. Canter GJ, De la Torre R, Mier M (1961) A method for evaluating disability in patients with Parkinson's Disease. J Nerv Ment Dis 122: 143–147
4. Freed CR, Breeze RE, Rosenberg NL *et al* (1990) Transplantation of human fetal dopamine cells for Parkinson's disease: Results at one year. Arch Neurol 47: 505–512
5. Hitchcock ER, Kenny BG, Clough CG, Hughes RC, Henderson BTH, Detta A (1990) Stereotactic implantation of Foetal Mesesencephalon (STIM): The UK experience. In: Dunnett SB, Richards SJ (eds) Neural transplantation: from molecular basis to clinical applications. Prog Brain Res 82: 723–728 Elsevier, Amsterdam, New York, Oxford
6. Lindvall O, Rehncrona S, Brundin P *et al* (1989) Human fetal dopamine neurons grafted into the Striatum in two patients with severe Parkinson's disease: a detailed account of methodology and a 6-month follow-up. Arch Neurol 46: 615–631
7. Nutt JG (1987) On-off Phenomenon: Relation to Levodopa Pharmacokinetics and Pharmacodynamics. Ann Neurol 22: 535–540
8. Perlow MJ, Freed WJ, Hoffer BJ *et al* (1979) Brain grafts reduce motor abnormalities produced by destruction of nigrostriatal dopamine system. Science 204: 643–647
9. Sladek JR Jr, Redmond DE Jr, Collier TJ *et al* (1987) Transplantation of fetal dopamine neurons in primate brain reverses MPTP induced parkinsonism. Prog Brain Res 71: 309–323
10. Webster DD (1968) Critical analysis of the disability in Parkinson's disease. Mod Treat 5: 257–282

Correspondence: B.T.H. Henderson, Department of Neurosurgery, University of Birmingham, Midland Centre for Neurosurgery and Neurology, Smethwick, Birmingham, UK.

Acta Neurochirurgica, Suppl. 52, 51–53 (1991)

Grafting of Fetal Dopamine Neurons in Parkinson's Disease The Czech Experience with Severe Akinetic Patients

O. Subrt, M. Tichy[1], **V. Vladyka,** and **K. Hurt**[2]

Departments of Neurosurgery, [1]Child Neurosurgery and [2]Gynecology and Obstetrics, Charles University Medical Schools, Prague, Czech and Slovak Federative Republic

Summary

Preliminary results in three patients with Parkinson's disease, who had transplantation of human embryonic mesencephalic tissue into the caput nuclei caudati, are reported. Some improvement was achieved.

Keywords: Parkinson's disease; transplantation; human embryonic mesencephalic tissue; nucleus caudatus; results.

Introduction

Neural transplantation was initially perceived as an experimental tool for the systematic study of neural development and regeneration, particularly in invertebrate species where regenerative capacities are most robust. Initial examination of this question in mammals invariably relied upon the same rationale, but this shifted dramatically when several groups of investigators discovered that a variety of neurological deficits could be improved with neural grafting, particularly if the donor cells were derived from fetal brain. The possible clinical application of neural grafting in patients with Parkinson's disease was first suggested a decade ago when it was reported that striatal implants of dopaminergic ventral mesencephalic tissue from fetuses could reduce symptoms of Parkinsonian syndrome in rats or non human primates induced by 6-hydroxydopamine or methyl-phenyl-tetrahydropyridine /MPTP/.

We have also a relatively large group of neurophysiologists who have an interest in neurotransplantation in the Czechoslovak Academy of Science. From this group came the first proposal of clinical applications of fetal implantations. We tried out this method on rats and monkeys and last year we prepared the first human operations. We now have more than one year of experience with follow up of these patients after implantation.

We describe some preliminary information about our method, indication criteria, results and the changes of our methodology after these first experience. Our method attempts to reduce exogenous influences on the implant tissue. Since we do not have sufficient information about the mechanisms of tissue implants effects we have to protect not only the neurones, but also the glial cells and the natural relation of these elements. This is particularly relevant if the trophic theory of growth factors from fetal tissue is now the most probable. It justifies the use of tissue blocks and no suspension of cells without application of immunosupression.

Methods

In three patients implantation of mesencephalic tissue from 7–8 weeks old human embryos into the caput nuclei caudati has been done. Fetal tissue was obtained from elective abortion; before abortion we test the donor for virus infections [HIV, CMV, hepatitis B virus]. The abortions were done by aspiration with low pressure pump and transparent cannula after the small dilatation of cervical canal maximal to Number 12 Hegar dilator.

Fetuses are transported in a sterile isotonic glucose-saline solution and the tissue is prepared at the neurosurgery department. Preparation was done under the operating microscope [Opton-Zeiss 6], with magnification about 15 times. After removing meninges we dissected the ventral part of mesencephalon. This tissue was cut into 3 or 4 pieces and gently sucked into the cannula. After the dissection the close piece of mesencephalic tissue is taken for bacterial examination and histological evaluation.

The small tissue blocks were implanted stereotactically into the head of the caudate nucleus unilaterally through the frontal burr hole. The implantations were carried out on the side contralateral to the worse parkinsonian's symptoms. A specially constructed instrument, consisting of an outer cannula with mandrin and an inner canula was used for the implantations. The outer diameter of the outer cannula was 2.2 mm and of the inner one 1.6 mm. Mandrin of the outer cannula is longer to prepare the bed for the tissue pieces. Fetal tissue was introduced to the target point in the inner cannula. This procedure was performed under local anesthesia. Implantation was completed to 3 hours after abortion. We gave before operation and one day after antibiotics [Cęfamezin] as bacterial prophylaxis.

The patients continued to receive the same doses of parkinsonian medication after the operation, but later the L-dopa doses were adjusted according to clinical status. We have followed the patients for 3, 6, 9 months and 1 year. We evaluated clinical status by functional tests with videorecoding, EEC, neurohormones level in the CSF and MRI. The functional tests we performed after a 14 hours period without exogenous L-Dopa.

Results

The first improvement of the parkinsonian's symptoms we saw after three months. Our patients stated from the first a prolongation of the ON interval after the administration of L-dopa and earlier start of the favorable reaction. Later the patients were relived of L-dopa side-effects and could reduce the daily dosage. Daily dosage of L-dopa and duration of ON effect without hyperkinetic side-effects are shown in the figures (Figs. 1 and 2). The relative best improving we observed on the second patient. This woman had a very severe akinetic form of Parkinson's disease. Some months before operation she only lay in bed, and had to be fed and often had to be in hospital, because only intravenous administration of anticholinergic drugs could alleviate the symptoms of parkinsonian's crisis. Now she could eat alone, walk with a stick and the implantation changed the quality of her life.

Further two patients have also shown improvement of the L-dopa effect since we could reduce the daily dosage to 60%. The functional test on the videorecording improved about 20%. Also the first patient, now 18 month after implantation, has returned to work. However these patients do not value their improvement very highly. There were small changes in Hoehn/Yahr stages of his disease before and after

Table 1. *Results. 3 Patients (Two After 1 Year, one After 8 Month)*

- good improvement of hypokinesia
- intensity of tremor without changes
- removal of Parkinsonian crisis
  (the 2nd patient with hard vegetative signs)
- the first signs of improvement in the end of the 2nd month after implantation
- initial dose of L-dopa provokes after the half year signs of overdose, reduction of initial dose to 2/3–1/2
- conspicuous symptoms of improvement are prolongation of daily walk and time of good condition

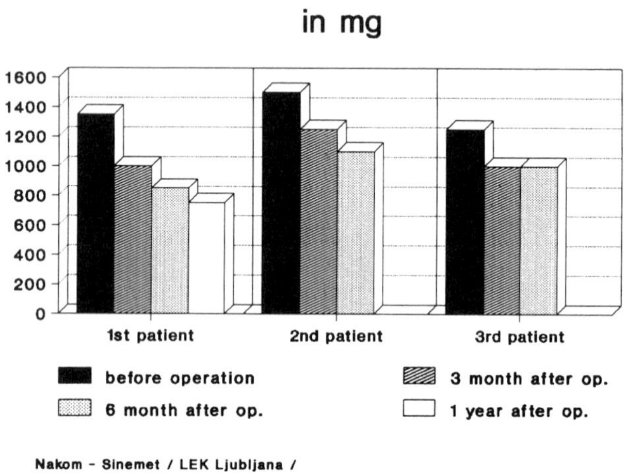

Fig. 1. Daily dosage of L-dopa

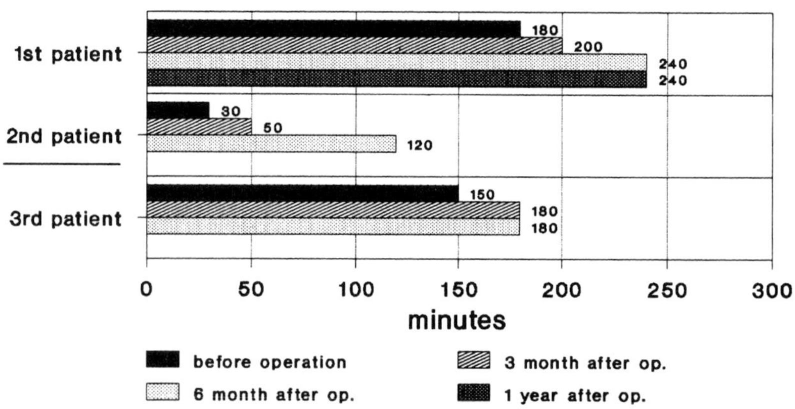

Fig. 2. Duration of "good" condition after 250 mg L-dopa (Nakom)

the implantation. The special function tests [pronation/supination test, simple and complex arm and hand movements tests or finger test] are good for scientific studies of this problem, but if the quality of life does not expressively change, the patient does not feel the therapy is successful. That is why we now select for this operation patients with severe akinesis, in H/Y stage IV or V.

In this time we changed our method of the fetal tissue preservation. According to experiences of the Florida's transplantation group and also others the fetal brain tissue is not so tender and lives in vitro longer than we believed. We now use a special saline solution with glucose and lactic acid and can preserve the tissue pieces from three to five days in temperature from 4 to 6 degree. The results of other groups encourages to implant the mesencephalic tissue to more targets in the caudate nucleus and putamen.

Correspondence: O. Subrt, Department of Neurosurgery, 1st School of Medicine, Charles University, CS-169 02, UVN-Stresovice, Prague 6, Czechoslovakia.

Acta Neurochirurgica, Suppl. 52, 54–57 (1991)

A Series of Experimental Surgery for Advanced Parkinson's Disease by Foetal Mesencephalic Transplantation

E.R. Hitchcock, B.G. Kenny, B.T.H. Henderson, C.G. Clough, R.C. Hughes, and **A. Detta**

Department of Neurosurgery, University of Birmingham, Midland Centre for Neurosurgery and Neurology, Smethwick, Birmingham, U.K.

Summary

12 patients with advanced Parkinson's Disease who had right caudate implantations of late stage foetal mesencephalon have been followed up for 1 to 2 years with extensive clinical and physiological assessments. Three patients failed to comply and were excluded. Seven of the remaining 9 patients showed substantial initial improvement which was well maintained in 4. Two of the 3 remaining patients of this group maintained lesser improvement. One returned to pre-operative state. Two patients with greatly advanced disease had only slight but brief improvement.

A series of 24 matched patients have been treated and continue under investigation.

Keywords: Parkinson's disease; transplantation, foetal Mesencephalon.

Introduction

The laboratory basis for clinical transplantation has been extensively reviewed[10,11,21]. Despite the great species difference the important first steps in our understanding of the requirements for successful clinical transplantation were established in rodent models. Increasing importance is attributed to the less extensive but more relevant investigations in non-human primates[1,2,3,8,16,19].

Clinical experiments have conformed to either rodent or non-human primate experience. Lindvall's[12] group who have made significant contributions to our basic understanding have consistently followed their laboratory practice so that material is from the first trimester, disaggregated and trypsinised and immunosuppression is used. Madrazo[13] and Molina[14] however, used solid fragments of first trimester with immunosuppression, whilst Freed using first trimester material used immunosuppression in one patient but not in another[7].

Non-human primate studies of Sladek[20] suggests that foetuses older than the first trimester may be used without immunosuppression. A pilot study (Series 1)[10] has been completed in patients with Hoehn and Yahr Stage IV-V PD who had stereotactic implantation of mid-trimester foetal mesencephalon into the head of the right caudate nucleus without immunosuppression. We have now followed up all these patients for more than one year[9]. The severity of Parkinson's Disease in different operative series is often difficult to establish, and described in different ways and is both variable between and within the same groups; investigation and assessment has been similarly variable.

Method

This first series confirmed the protean nature of advanced Parkinson's Disease and the resultant difficulties in producing consistently quantifiable assessments. Because of the experimental nature of the treatment we selected patients with advanced PD. Full Ethical Committee approval was given and the protocol conformed to ethical guidelines[15].

Our clinical series was designed to determine whether the non-human primate findings can be confirmed in man. We attempted to minimise experimental variables by controlling the following factors. (i) A single striatal site: avoids uncertainties of multiple site implantations and facilitates detection of ipsi or contralateral effects. (ii) Single mid trimester foetus: to avoid the uncertainties of multiple genomes. This permitted sufficient body fluid to test for infective agents such as HIV and cytomegalovirus, Hepatitis B and HSV. (iii) No immunosuppression: Non-human primate allografts survived successfully without immunosuppression (Sladek[20] and the hazards of immuno-suppression in man are well known (iv) Clump implantation: Complete cellular disaggregation damages the more mature cell[17] while solid masses may succumb to the effects of ischaemia. Clumps of human third trimester mesencephalic cells retain better viability when mechanically disaggregated than when enzymatically dispersed[6].

The method of foetal harvesting has been described elsewhere[10]. The whole procedure is performed under local anaesthesia thus permitting serial neurological assessment. Following application of the stereotactic square the target is chosen from CT images after reference to stereotactic brain atlases and the images reformatted to produce visualisation of the target and planned trajectory. An implantation cannula (OD 0.9 mm. ID 0.5 mm.) is directed to the target site. After radiological confirmation of correct position the specimen is slowly injected. The patient is fully ambulant on the first post-operative day.

Results

Series 1: Consisted of 9 males and 3 females aged 41 to 67 years. Extensive pre- and post-operative clinical and physiological assessments were made at 1, 3, 6, 9 and 12 month intervals. Three patients unable to comply with the follow-up protocol were excluded from the trial. Seven of 9 patients showed substantial initial improvement well maintained in 4. (Fig. 1). Of the remaining three patients two maintained a lesser improvement and one returned to his pre-operative state. Two patients with the most advanced disease had only slight and brief improvement before resuming their pre-operative decline.

Series 2 and 3: Two further series have been completed and the results are now undergoing analysis. 12 patients (Series 2) received right putaminal implantations and were matched against 12 patients (Series 3) who were used as controls until they received a right caudate head implantation and acted thereafter as their own controls.

Discussion

Laboratory experiments have shown that disaggregation is harmful to foetal cells[5] which may be due to the fragility of processes arising from the developing mature neurones. Many of the injected cells are still in the proliferative phase although we are not yet able to determine their particular cell type. Cells may be injured during passage through the stereotactic implantation cannula; fully dispersed foetal cells are more vulnerable to narrow needle passage than cell clumps. The reason for the comparative failure of human foetal cell xenografts to rodents may be related to the method of tissue preparation[6].

We come now to an important conceptual problem. Animal studies suggest that mitotic or pre-mitotic dopaminergic cells should be implanted in the hope that continued division would increase their number. Similarly, complete disaggregation was initiated to encourage dispersion of cells[4]. The evidence is that disaggregated embryonic cells will disperse but little to suggest that these proliferate; on that basis, sufficient cells must be implanted to replace the degenerate cells. In first trimester implantation this can only be achieved by using several foetal specimens in each patient[12]. There are considerable logistical clinical problems in obtaining sufficient specimens at one time.

An almost universal finding in clinical studies throws doubt on these simplistic concepts; in strictly unilateral dopamine cell implantations a bilateral

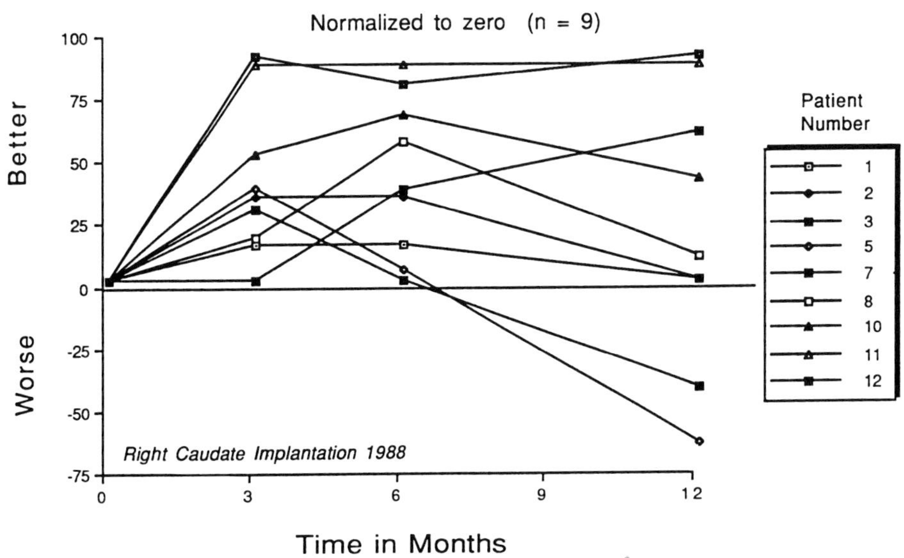

Fig. 1.

Table 1. *Neural Transplantation Protocol*

Clinical

- General description physical state/diagnostic confirmation
- Drug dosage
- Subjective definition and description of "on" and "off"
- Hoehn and Yahr, WRS, NUDS, UPDRS, and ADL
- Timed motor response/ambulation
- Standard L-Dopa response test

Foetal

- Age: post concept/US/crown rump/development
- Sex
- Time/date termination
- Tissue type. Donor and recipient
- Dissection method/volume material
- Virology

Surgery

- Time last dose medication
- Stereo instrument/target method
- X-ray confirmation cannula position

Post-operative management

- Optimal post-operative medication. 3, 6, 12 months regular assessment

effect is usually demonstrable inexplicable by theories of proliferation or synaptic connection. The possibility of some "factor" other than dopamine must be considered[3].

If we are to benefit from these investigations and proceed with our clinical studies we must try to adopt some consistent method of reporting our results and we suggest the following protocol (Table 1). If we are to engage in this experimental treatment and are necessarily uncertain how much good we can do we must certainly strive to avoid doing harm. The use of stereotactic methods are the most reliable, scientific and the least traumatic.

Acknowledgements

BTHH is Parkinsons Disease Society Research Fellow.

References

1. Bakay RAE, Fiandaca MS, Barrow DL, Schiff A, Collins DC (1985) Preliminary report on the use of fetal tissue transplantation to correct MPTP-induced Parkinson like syndrome in primates. Appl Neurophysiol 48: 358–361
2. Bankiewiez KS, Jacobowitz DM, Plunkett RJ, Oldfield EH, Kopin J (1987) Injury induced sprouting into the caudate nucleus, after solid tissue implantation in MPTP-induced Parkinsonism monkeys. Soc Neurosci Abstract 36: 16
3. Bankiewiez KS, Jacobowitz DM, Plunkett RJ, Oldfield EH, Kopin IJ Fetal non-dopaminergic neural implants in Parkinsonian Primates: Histochemical and behavioural studies. J Neurosurg (in press)
4. Bjorklund A, Stenevi U, Schmidt RH, Dunnett SB, Gage FH (1983) Intracerebral grafting of neuronal cell suspensions. I. Introduction and general methods of preparation. II. Survival and growth of nigral cell suspensions implanted in different brain sites. Acta Physiol Scan [Suppl] 522: 1–18
5. Detta A, Hitchcock ER (1990) The selective viability of human foetal brain cells. Brain Res 520: 277–283.
6. Detta A, Hitchcock ER (1991) Influence of needle lumen size on viability of injected dispersed and clumped foetal brain cells. Restorative Neurol and Neurosci 2: 77–80
7. Freed CR, Breeze RE, Rosenberg NL *et al* (1990) Therapeutic effects of human fetal dopamine cells transplanted in a patient with Parkinson's Disease. In: Dunnett SB, Richards SJ (eds) Neural transplantation: From molecular basis to clinical applications Elsevier Amsterdam, New York, Oxford. Prog Brain Res 82: 715–721
8. Freed CR, Richards JB, Hutt C, Whalen J, Peterson R, Reite M (1987) Behavioral effects of fetal dopamine cell transplantation in bonnet monkeys with MPTP – induced Parkinsonism. Soc Neurosci Abstract 219: 5
9. Henderson BTH, Clough CG, Hughes RC, Hitchcock ER, Kenny BG Implantation of Human Fetal Ventral Mesencephalon to the Right Caudate Nucleus in Advanced Parkinson's Disease. Arch Neurol (in press)
10. Hitchcock ER, Kenny BG, Clough CG, Hughes RC, Henderson BTH, Detta A (1990) Stereotactic implantation of foetal mesencephalon (STIM): The UK Experience. In: Dunnett SB, Richards SJ (eds) Neural Transplantation: from molecular basis to clinical applications. Elsevier, Amsterdam, New York, Oxford. Prog Brain Res 82: 723–728
11. Lindvall O (1989) Transplantation into the human brain: present status and future possibilities. Neurology, Neurosurgery and Psychiatry Special Supplement 39–54
12. Lindvall O, Rehncrona S, Brundin P *et al* (1989) Human fetal dopamine neurones grafted into the striatum in two patients with severe Parkinson's Disease. Arch Neurol 46: 615–631
13. Madrazo I, Leon V, Torres C *et al* (1988) Transplantation of fetal substantia nigra and adrenal medulla to the caudate nucleus in two patients with Parkinson's Disease. New Engl J Med 318: 51
14. Molina H *et al* (1989) Neurotransplantation in Parkinson's Disease – the Cuban experience. In: Neural Transplantation: From molecular basis to clinical application. Restorative Neurology and Neuroscience [Suppl] 230:
15. Review of the Guidance on the Research Use of Fetuses and Fetal Material. Report of the Polkinghorne Commission. (1979) HMSO CM 762
16. Redmond DEJ Jr, Sladek JR Jr, Roth RH *et al* (1986) Fetal neuronal grafts in monkeys given methylphenyltetrahydropyridine. Lancet i: 1125–1127
17. Schmidt RH, Bjorklund A, Stenevi U (1981) Intracerebral grafting of dissociated CNS tissue suspensions. A new approach for neuronal transplantation to deep brain sites. Brain Res 218: 347–356
18. Sladek JR, Collier JJ, Haber SN, Roth RH, Redmond E (1986) Survival and growth of foetal catecholamine neurones transplanted into primate brain. Brain Res Bulletin 17: 809–818
19. Sladek JR Jr, Redmond E, Collier TJ, Blount JP, Elsworth JD, Taylor JR, Roth RH (1988) In: Gash DM, Sladek JR Jr (eds) Transplantation in Mammalian CNS. Fetal dopamine grafts

extended reversal of methylphenyltetrahydropyridine-induced Parkinsonism in monkeys. Prog Brain Res 78: 497–506
20. Sladek JR, Redmond DE, Collier TJ, Haber SN, Elsworth JD, Deutsch AY, Roth RH (1987) Transplantation of fetal dopamine neurons in primate brain reverses MPTP-induced Parkinsonism. (eds) FJ Seil, E Herbert, BM Carlson. Elsevier Science Publications BV, Biomedical Division. Prog Brain Res 71: 309–323
21. Sladek JR, Gash DM (1988) Nerve cell-grafting in Parkinson's Disease. J Neurosurg 68: 337–351

Correspondence: E.R. Hitchcock, Department of Neurosurgery, University of Birmingham, Midland Centre for Neurosurgery and Neurology, Holly Lane Smethwick, Birmingham B67 7JX, U.K.

Technical Contributions

Acta Neurochirurgica, Suppl. 52, 61–63 (1991)

Digital X-Ray Apparatus Especially Designed for Precise Biometry in Stereotactic Surgical Procedures

F. Giunta and **C. Gilardoni**[1]

Neurosurgery, University of Brescia, Spedali Civili, Brescia and [1]Gilardoni's Research Laboratories, Mandello Lario, Como, Italy

Summary

Modern stereotactic surgical procedures were developed mainly because digital CT image gave us the opportunity to recognize the morphology and the site of a brain lesion, and, at the same time, CT offered a very easy and reliable way to calculate target coordinates because the brain scans are digital maps. Digital x-ray image obtained with an x-ray-intensifier and a TV Analog/Digital converter is not suitable for stereotactic use because image distortion is multifactorial and it is impossible to rectify.

We have developed a new apparatus (Neurogil) for intra-operative use that is able to produce a digital image on a display, the measures displayed match exactly with the patient's brain. A linear array of 1024 photodiodes is working in front of an x-ray source and it collects the density image of the patient's head positioned between them. It shows the patient's head with the stereotactic frame exactly as a radiogram, but no distortion is present. Digital brain angiograms are possible with electronic subtraction, mathematical enhancement and with a stereoscopic view on a particular display. Any kind of mathematical calculation or computer-graphic application is possible. A special software was developed for stereotactic closed and open surgery.

Keywords: Digital x-ray apparatus; biometry; stereotactic neurosurgery.

Introduction

Before CT era the stereotactic neurosurgery was developed around the possibility to visualize some brain structures on x-ray films and to calculate brain structures not seen on x-ray films using brain maps. All operative rooms dedicated to stereotactic surgery had x-ray apparatus to take images. The problem was the enlargement of x-ray image because of a conic projection of x-ray from the source to the film. Measures were taken manually and calculations were in some manner time consuming during the surgical procedure. But x-ray apparatus in operative room offered the possibility to take angiograms in stereotactic conditions and take control pictures during the surgical procedure. This was a very important surgical tool and safety was obtained.

The modern stereotactic surgical procedure is mainly due to the possibility to visualize patient's brain in digital images by those obtained with Computerized Tomography (CT) or Magnetic Resonance (MR). Their images give the opportunity to recognize exactly the site and the extension of any brain lesion and, at the same time, offer a very easy and reliable way to calculate the target points because the brain scans are digital maps exactly corresponding to patient's brain. Only at the Digital Angiography (DA) measures do not correspond to the living brain because x-ray-intensifier and analogical to digital conversion introduces a number of distortions impossible to rectify (Fig. 1).

With CT and MR digital images is so easy to take true measures that a number of computer aided tools were developed to simulate stereotactic surgery, give spatial coordinates, calculate volumes of cysts or isodoses for the brachitherapy and match with brain maps for functional surgery[2,3,4,5,7,8,15,17,19]. These features make stereotaxis easy. But often it is useful to verify the surgical procedure and an intra-operative control is mandatory mainly if, together with the lesion, the vascular tree is necessary to visualize.

The opportunity to plan and verify stereotactic procedure step by step during surgery, without limit to any surgical approach (convexity, temporal or cerebellar), and to obtain serial angiograms in stereotactic conditions with x-ray digital images computer generated, coherent with the patient's brain, was the target of our research.

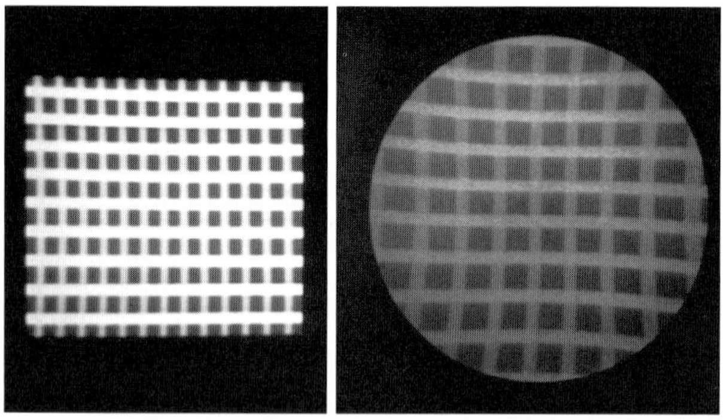

Fig. 1. (a) Digital radiography of an orthogonal net taken with an x-ray-intensifier and a TV analog to digital converter. Line and angles are not orthogonal. Distortion is not possible to correct mathematically. (b) First experimental digital image with Neurogil. The same net. It is possible to take images of larger subjects. Line and angles are exactly orthogonal.

Material and Methods

Equipment Description

We have developed a new equipment (Neurogil) for intra-operative use that is able to give a digital-x-ray image on a display and the biological measures match exactly the patient's brain.

The Neurogil is on a steel ring, hanging from the operative room roof or on reels, is moving all around the patient's head and its diameter allow an adequate brain surgical approach contemporary with images taking. It carries an x-ray source and, in the opposite side, a detector array. Patient's head is positioned in the middle of the ring. X-ray source and detector are able to rotate freely all around the patients's head in every plane needed with robotized movements.

Detector is an array of 1024 photodiodes working in front of the x-ray source to produce a digital image with 1024 × 1024 pixels displayed on a CRT. It shows the patient's head with the stereotactic frame like a radiogram do, but no distortion is present and any computer manipulation is possible: for calculations, electronic image subtraction, mathematical enhancement and computer graphic elaborations. It is possible to take stereoscopic views in any projection.

Neurogil is a computerized x-ray equipment and there are two computer console. The system console, with three monitor (one to talk with the computer and two with graphic images and pop-up menues of a dedicated software), controls the whole x-ray equipment and digital images. It is working in a room adjacent to operative room. Into the operative room there is the surgical console with two monitors and a sterilized mouse that allows the surgeon to talk with the computer to take images and elaborate them.

Digital brain serial Angiograms are obtained with or without stereoscopic view in stereotactic conditions. Automatic electronic subtraction and computer graphic are possible. Wessels over 0.5 mm are displayed because pixels are 0.45 mm.

A special software was developed for stereotactic close and open surgery.

The ionizing dose given to the patient's head is very low because the subject is scanned by the beam and not totally irradiated.

Surgical Procedure

Surgery starts with the application of the stereotactic frame to the patient's head, usually in neuroleptoanalgesia. A CT or MR is done to visualize brain lesions and stereotactic frame, so exact calculations and matching with Neurogil images are possible. CT or MR images are transferred from Radiology to Operative Room by a LAN and are stored into Neurogil's computer like a 3D array, so reconstruction in any plane is possible. In operative room a digital angiography in stereotactic conditions is done to analize the vascularity of the lesion and surgery is accomplished with step by step control. Intraoperative control is necessary during high risk biopsies, bulk removals, isotope implants in solid or cystic tumors. In functional neurosurgery ventriculography is mandatory to exact visualization of classical parameters.

Discussion

Computer aided stereotactic surgery has created so many electronic tools that it seems that intraoperative controls are not necessary[15,19]. Sometime it is true, but in many surgical procedures intraoperative controls are mandatory and no surgery is possible without them. On the other hand no surgical x-ray equipment was recently designed with modern features to interfacing with the computerized radiology. The "therapeutic CT"[11,12,13,18] is a good solution, but not optimal, because it do not show the vascular tree (very important for surgical safety) and reduces surgical approaches.

Digital x-ray image obtained with an x-ray-intensifier and a TV A/D converter is not suitable for stereotactic use because image distortion is multi-factorial and it is impossible to rectify (Fig. 1).

The ultrasonography in operative room[1,9,10,14,15] does not belong to a stereotactic tool because there are no spatial coordinates, but one can use for a visual direct control like CT guided procedures. In addition ultrasonography is safe if mass lesion is large enough (over 1.5 cm) and not too deeply seated[16].

The neurophysiological control is mandatory in functional neurosurgery, but ventriculography is always the most important tool during surgery, together with CT or MR brain images.[1,6].

References

1. Asakura T, Uetsuhara K, Kanemaru R, Hirahara K (1985) An applicability study on a CT-guided stereotactic technique for functional neurosurgery. Appl Neurophysiol 48: 73–76
2. Brown FD, Rachlin JR, Rubin JM, Fessler RG, Smith LJ, Schaible KL (1984) Ultrasound-guided periventricular stereotaxis. Neurosurgery 15: 162–164
3. Clarke L (1988) Computer assisted stereotactic surgery. Can Oper Room Nurs J 6: 14–24
4. Froeder M, Seitzer D, Buren G, Dieckmann G (1983) Digital Radiography for target point evaluation in stereotactic neurosurgery. Appl Neurophysiol 46: 206–210
5. Goodman JH, Watkins ES, Davis JR, Mullin BB (1987) Microcomputer stereotactic atlas. Appl Neurophysiol 50: 6

6. Hadley MN, Shetter AG, Amos MR (1985) Use of the Brown-Roberts-Wells stereotactic frame for functional neurosurgery. Appl Neurophysiol 48: 61–68
7. Jenny AB, Biondetti PR, Layton B, Knapp RH (1988) The computer and stereotactic surgery in neurological surgery. Comput Med Imaging Graph 12: 75–83
8. Kall BA, Kelly PJ, Goerss SJ (1986) The computer as a stereotactic surgical instrument. Neurol Res 8: 201–208
9. Knake JE, Chandler WF, Gabrielsen TO, Latack JT, Gebraski SS (1984) Intraoperative sonography delineation of low-grade brain neoplasms defined poorly by computed tomography. Radiology 151: 735–739
10. Koivukangas J, Kelly PJ (1986) Application of ultrasound imaging to stereotactic brain tumor surgery. Ann Clin Res 47: 25–32
11. Lunsford LD (1982) A dedicated CT system for the stereotactic operating room. Appl Neurophysiol 45: 374–378
12. Lunsford LD, Nelson PB (1982) Stereotactic aspiration of a brain abscess using a "therapeutic" CT scanner. Acta Neurochir (Wien) 62: 25–29
13. Lunsford LD, Rosenbaum AE, Perry J (1982) Stereotactic surgery using the "therapeutic" CT scanner. Surg Neurol 18: 116–122
14. Masuzawa H, Kanazawa I, Kamitani H, Sato J (1985) Intraoperative ultrasonography through a burr-hole. Acta Neurochir (Wien) 77: 41–45
15. Peters TM, Olivier A, Bertrand G (1983) The role of computed tomographic and digital radiographic techniques in stereotactic procedures for electrode implantation and mapping, and lesion localization. Appl Neurophysiol 46: 200–205
16. Roux FX, Ben Simon JL, Rey A, George B, Melki JP, Reizine D, Cophignon J (1983) Utilisation de l'ultrasonographie en temps reel en neurochirurgie. Interet per-operatoire chez l'adulte. Neurochirurgie 29: 31–35
17. Ten Haken RK, Diaz RF, McShan DL, Fraass BA, Taren JA, Hood TW (1988) From manual to 3-D computerized treatment plannin for 125-I stereotactic brain implants. Int J Radiat Oncol Biol Phys 15: 467–480
18. Uematsu S, Rosenbaum AE, Erozan YS, Gupta PK, Moses H, Nauta HJ, Rigsby WH, Wang A, Weiderman L, Kumar AJ (1987) Intraoperative CT monitoring during stereotactic brain surgery. Acta Neurochir (Wien) [Suppl] 39: 18–20
19. Watanabe E, Watanabe T, Manaka S, Mayanagi Y, Takakura K (1987) Three-dimensional digitizer (neuronavigator): New equipment for computed tomography-guided stereotaxic surgery. Surg Neurol 27: 543–547

Correspondence: F. Giunta, Neurosurgery, University of Brescia, Spedali Civili, Brescia, Italy.

Acta Neurochirurgica, Suppl. 52, 64–66 (1991)

An Ultrasound-Guided Stereotactic Apparatus for Intracranial Mass Lesions

H. Kawabatake, K. Amano, H. Kawamura, T. Tanikawa, H. Iseki, Y. Iwata, T. Taira, T. Shimizu, Y. Umezawa, K. Arai, and **H. Kawasaki**

Department of Neurosurgery, Neurological Institute, Tokyo Women's Medical College, Tokyo, Japan

Summary

One of disadvantages of conventional stereotactic operation for intracranial mass lesions is that it is basically a blind procedure even if the operation is performed in a gantry of a CT scan. High resolution ultrasound image gives real-time information on intracranial pathology such as bleeding, remaining cyst fluid or haematoma. The authors report an ultrasound guided stereotactic apparatus which gives real-time images of the lesion during operation.

Keywords: Ultrasound image; stereotaxis; real-time image.

Introduction

The recent development of ultrasound image technology has greatly improved the quality of imaging intracranial structures. Unfortunately its image is still not as good as those of computed tomography and magnetic resonance image. The main advantage of ultrasound image however is that it gives real-time information and even visualizes moving objects.

The conventional image-guided streotactic operation utilizes plain x-ray, CT scan and MR image. These images are not real-time in its true sense and the operation is basically a blind procedure even if it is performed in a CT gantry.

The authors made an ultrasound-guided stereotactic apparatus for intracranial mass lesions. Once an appropriate target is chosen on the ultrasound image, a needle for biopsy or drainage is precisely introduced to the target. Motion of the needle and changes of the intracranial lesion such as minor bleeding or decreasing volume of a cyst are visualized on the image.

Description of the Apparatus

The ultrasound probe is a pencil-shaped sector type 14 mm in diameter (Toshiba) and is attached to the stereotactic device. The stereotactic device consists of the probe holder, needle guide and retractor attachment. This device is so small that the whole system is secured on a burr hole with a self-retaining retractor (Fig. 1).

A cone-shaped intracranial area is visualized three-dimensionally by rotating the ultrasound probe. Once an appropriate target is chosen, one can measure the distance between the target and the zero-point of the device on the display. Because the biopsy or aspiration needle is inserted at a fixed angle to the probe, the length of needle insertion required is calculated by the Pythagorean law (Fig. 2).

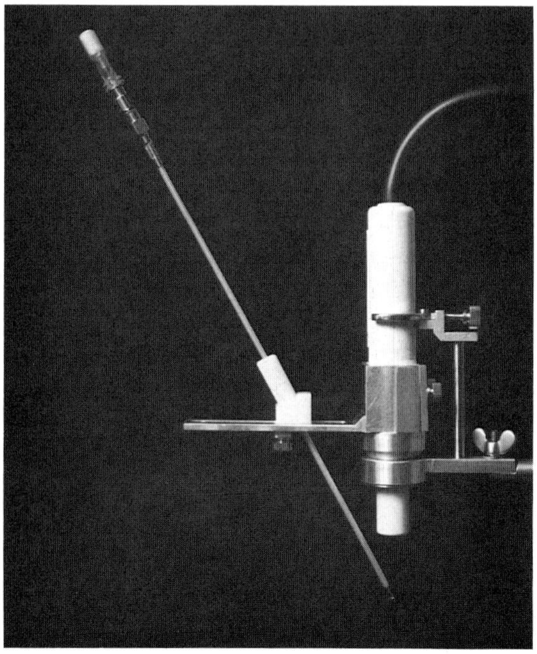

Fig. 1. Ultrasound probe and stereotactic device

Operative Procedure

The patient is placed on an operating table under either general or local anaesthesia. A burr hole is opened on the appropriate site and enlarged to about three centimeters in diameter. The dura is opened and the ultrasound probe attached to the stereotactic device is placed on the cortex. The direction of the probe is adjusted so that the lesion is well visualized. The device is then fixed with a self-retaining retractor. The distance between the zero-point of the device and the target is measured on the image. If the distance is 8 cm, the needle guide is slid 2 cm (8/4) from the zero-point. Because the zero-point is 2 cm from the centre of the probe, the length of the needle insertion is calculated as $(8^2+4^2)^{-2} = 8.94$ cm.

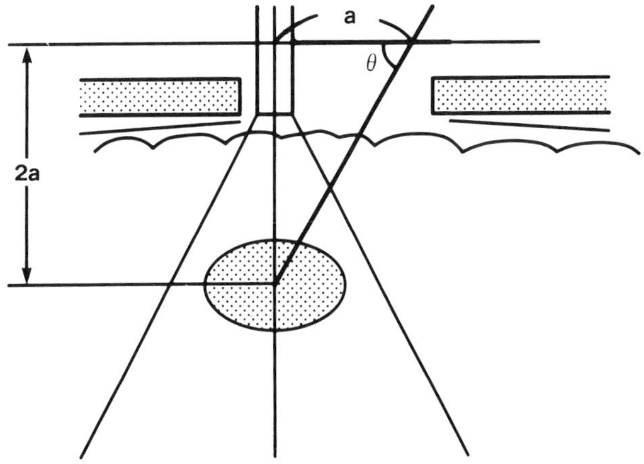

Fig. 2. Theory of target calculation

Discussion

The quality of the high resolution ultrasound image is sufficient to localize most intracranial lesions such as tumours, cysts and haematomas. Ventricles are also well visualized. There have been some reports on the utilization of intraoperative ultrasound images[1,2,3]. Some of them are, however, not truly stereotactic. The stereotactic device in the present report enables the surgeon to insert a needle precisely at the proposed target (Fig. 3). Unexpected bleeding from the biopsy site is well visualized and readily controlled. A cyst can be completely emptied, and even if another cyst is present and its location is moved by the first aspiration, it can be easily evacuated.

The disadvantage of ultrasound image is that it can not be applied over the skull. Therefore it is impossible to localize the appropriate site of the burr hole of craniotomy. Even if this disadvantage is taken into account, ultrasound-guided stereotactic surgery is useful for intracranial mass lesions.

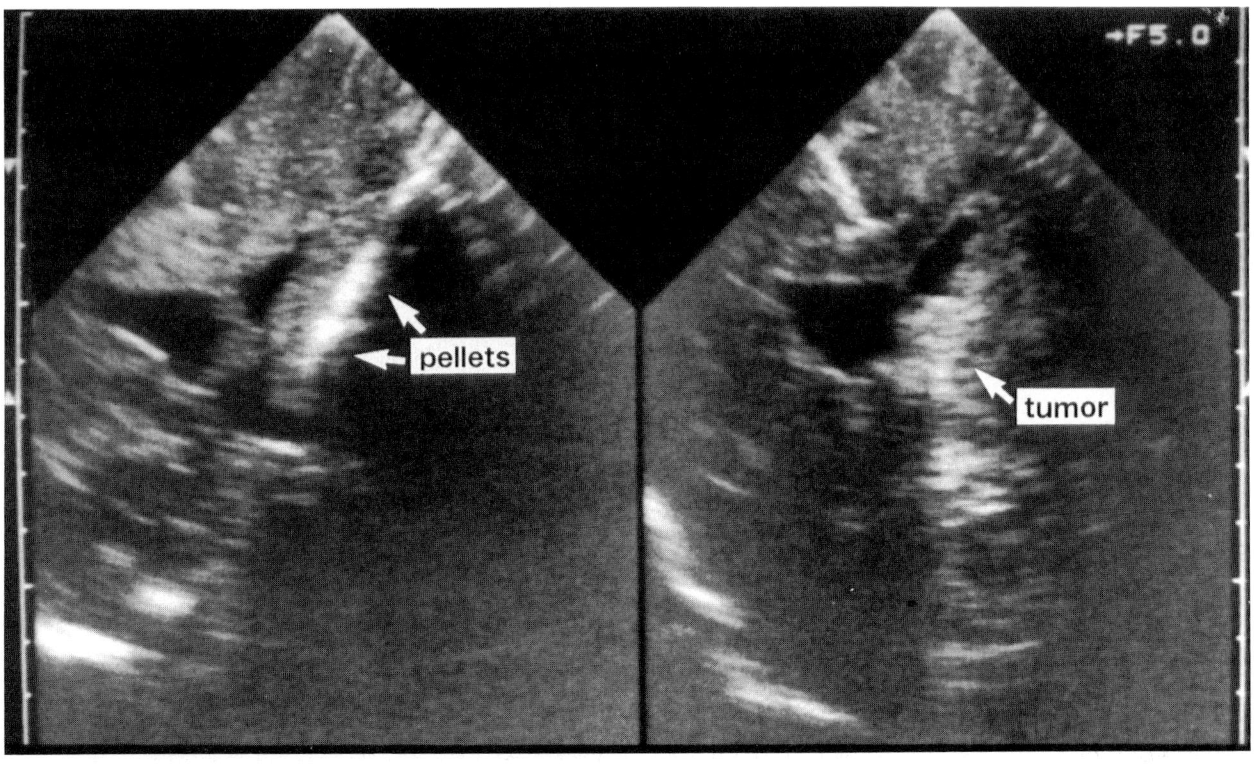

Fig. 3. Intra-tumoural implantation of pellets containing antitumour drug by ultrasound stereotaxis

References

1. Berger MS (1988) Ultrasound-guided stereotactic biopsy using a new apparatus. J Neurosurg 65: 550–554
2. Masuzawa H, Kamitani H, Sato J, Sakai F (1982) Intraoperative use of sector scanning ultrasonography in neurosurgery. Mod Neurosurg 1: 37–43
3. Tsutsumi Y, Andoh Y, Sakaguchi J (1989) A new ultrasound guided brain biopsy technique through a burr hole. Acta Neurochir (Wien) 96: 72–75

Correspondence: H. Kawabatake, Department of Neurosurgery, Neurological Institute, Tokyo Women's Medical College, Tokyo 162, Japan.

Acta Neurochirurgica, Suppl. 52, 67–68 (1991)

Application of Multimodality Imaging Stereotactic Localization in the Surgical Management of Vascular Lesions

L. Zamorano, B. Bauer-Kirpes, M. Dujovny, G. Malik, and **J. Ausman**

Henry Ford Neurosurgical Institute, Detroit, MI, USA

Summary

Multidimensional image preplanning and accurate pre and intraoperative localization for intracranial vascular lesions have been implemented. Methodology include carbon fiber base ring, localizer plates, any X-ray tubes, PC compatible software and intraoperative localizing unit. Surgical management of deep arteriovenous malformations is especially suitable for this technique, including the use of intraoperative digital angiography.

Keywords: Cerebro-vascular lesions; surgical management; multimodality imaging; stereotactic localization.

Introduction

Multidimensional image preplanning and accurate pre and intraoperative localization for intracranial vascular lesions have been implemented. Image data acquisition is performed with a CT, MRI and digital angiography compatible carbon fiber base ring. Tomographic data (CT, MRI) is used to perform 3D-2D surgical planning which include selection of surgical trajectory, characterization of vascular lesions "viewed" from different surgeons perspective. Four x-ray localizer plates are attached superior or inferior to the ring and angiographic studies are performed before, during and after surgery. The radiographs can be taken with any x-ray tubes including intraoperative digital angiography. Each plate has four landmarks which are the reference systems in AP and lateral films. Digitization of the reference landmarks and targets can be done on a digitizer tablet or using a camera and video-signal digital conversion hardware and software (frame grabber). Software has been implemented that calculates stereotactic coordinates of any desired target; the inverse is also possible: any target defined on tomographic images can be shown in the AP and lateral angiographic views. The system is indepehdent of angulation and film-focus distance. Intraoperative fully sterile conditions are accomplished with the localizing unit (ZD multipurpose localizing unit, Fisher, Freiburg, Germany) as well as unobstructed microsurgical approach. Intraoperative angiographic localization can be achieved with the positioned localizing unit also in sterile conditions; this becomes extremely useful in the intraoperative assessment of complete removal of deep arteriovenous malformations. Methodology, fundamentals and clinical examples are presented on this report.

Material and Method

Stereotactic x-ray Localization: In this report a method is described which allows the calculation of stereotactic target coordinates from two planar x-ray films. In contrary to other methods, such as teleradiography, it does not require:

- that the central beam is parallel to the ring axis
- that the films are orthogonal to the ring axis or to the central beam
- that distant x-ray source is used (standard film focus distance of less than 1 metre can be used)
- that radio-opaque scales are projected onto the films.

The present x-ray stereotactic localizing system consists of four plexiglass localizer plates with four markers on each, a digitizing tablet to measure the markers points or an image scanning system to import the x-ray films onto the computer screen and a PC compatible localizer software.

This x-ray stereotactic localizing system can be used for various stereotactic localization problems:

a) stereotactic coordinates of lesions such as arteriovenous malformations can be determined from two x-ray films
b) any probe (biopsy forceps, electrodes, cannula, etc) trajectroy can be verified during stereotactic surgery
c) the position of stereotactic I–125 seed implants can be verified during surgery
d) distances can be measured in x-ray films like the diameter of lesions.

With the same equipment and software the opposite functions can also be performed, i.e. to transfer CT or MRI coordinates into x-ray films:
a) stereotactic target points defined by CT or MRI can be localized into x-ray films;
b) before implanting a probe, its stereotactic trajectory can be projected on two x-ray films. Therefore, points can be identified that would intersect with vascular structures;
c) if the x-ray films have been scanned even target volume or isodose contours from treatment planning for interstitial radiotherapy or radiosurgery can be superimposed into x-ray images.

Fundamentals

Corresponding to the two classes of functions described above, two mathematical procedures have to be distinguished:
1. The transformation of film coordinates to stereotactic coordinates
2. The transformation of stereotactic coordinates to film coordinates
1. This procedure has already been described by other authors 1, 2. Various modifications of this method do exist and are based on the following principles: the two source targets rays intersect with the localizer plates at four points called A, P, L, R (Fig. 1). These points can be found by considering each plate independently. If these intersection points with the plates are calculated, the stereotactic coordinates of A, P, L, R can be easily determined. The lines A-P and L-R intersect in the target point which can then easily be calculated in stereotactic coordinates. If the lines do not intersect perfectly, the mid point of the shortest line segment connecting A-P and L-R is considered as the target point; the length of the line segment is displayed as "accuracy".

It remains to show how one of the points A-P. L-R can be calculated from the markers and the target point on the films. This is shown with the point R which is the intersection of the source target ray with the right localizer plate (Fig. 2). On an arbitrarily positioned film the four markers M1, M2, M3, M4 are projected with no sides parallel. By constructing the vanishing point of the

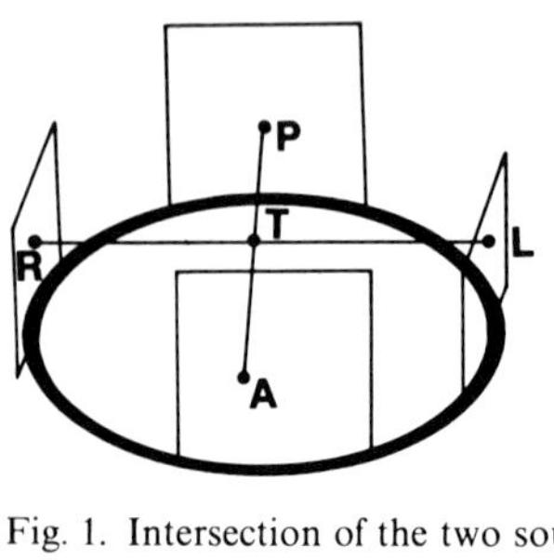

Fig. 1. Intersection of the two source-target rays with the localizer plates A, P, R, L

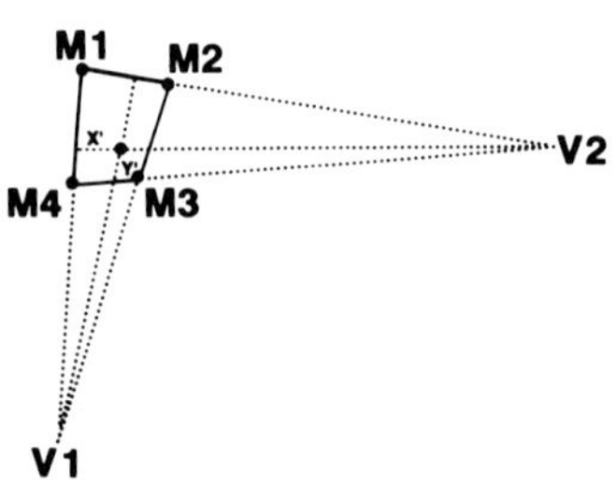

Fig. 2. Arbitrarily positioned film with four markers M1, M2, M3 and M4 projected with no sides parallel. By constructing V1 and V2 the coordinates of x′ and y′ relative to the square can be calculated

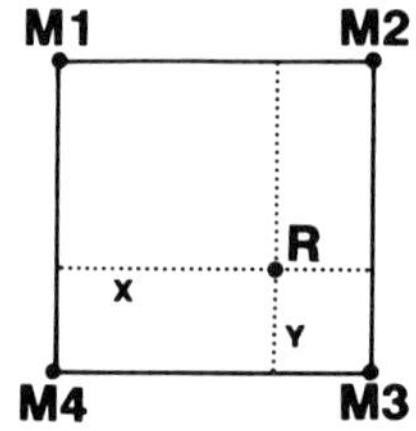

Fig. 3. Following the rules of perspective projection the stereotactic coordinates x′ and y′ can be calculated from x′ and y′

perspective projection V1 and V2 the coordinates of the target point ẋ and ẏ relative to the marker square can be calculated (Fig. 2). Following the rules of perspective projection the coordinates x and y can be calculated from x* and y* (Fig. 3).

The same formulas can also be applied if the target point on the films is not located within the rectangle made by the four markers. Then one or both of the target coordinates x, y is negative. Since the location of the four markers in the stereotactic coordinates system is known, the stereotactic coordinates of R can be calculated. The same procedure is repeated for the other localizer plates, giving the four points A, P, R, L.
2. The reverse projection of known stereotactic points onto the films uses the same information a procedure 1. Using the perspective transformation, the focus point of the lateral and AP x-ray source can be calculated in stereotactic space: With this information the transformation can be established in a 4x4 matrix. Then stereotactic coordinates of arbitrary points like target, entry point, contour points can be transformed into the two film coordinates system.

Discussion

A methodology has been presented that allows to localize targets into x-rays standard films. Stereotactic coordinates can be accurately obtained independently of x-ray-film distance or angulation. The reverse can also be accomplished i.e. the transfer of CT or MRI generated coordinates into x-ray films. The potential of the technique is highly useful in the management of vascular lesions including the stereotactic use of intraoperative digital angiography. Other uses include intraoperative verification of probes or seeds positioning, planning of stereotactic trajectories in relationship to vascular structures, etc. The potential of the technique is enormous for the three dimensional reconstruction of vascular structures based on tomographic and projective types of imaging.

References

1. Encarnacao J, Strasser W (1988) Computer graphics. Oldenburg, München
2. Siddon R, Barth N (1987) Stereotactic localization of intracranial targets. Int J Radiat Oncol Biol Phys 13: 1241–1246.

Correspondence: Lucia Zamorano, Henry Ford Neurosurgical Institute, 2799 West Grant Boulevard, Detroit, Michigan 48202–2689, USA.

Acta Neurochirurgica, Suppl. 52, 69–71 (1991)

Contemporary Stereotactic Atlasses: Merging of Functional Data with Individual Morphological MRI Acquisitions

C. Giorgi and **U. Cerchiari**[1]

Departments of Neurosurgery, Istituto Neurologico, [1]Computer Science, Ist. Naz dei Tumori, Milano, Italy

Summary

The traditional concept of the sterotactic brain atlas, utilized as an anatomical piece of information, to be integrated with neuroradiological data in order to organize functional observations, is evolving towards the creation of a powerful database for clinical and functional data, contained in anatomical structures. Actual computational resources make it possible to use this information, interactively adapted to each patient's anatomy, and updated, following each procedure.

Keywords: Stereotactic atlas: MRI; curvilinear matching; 3D matching.

Introduction

Traditional stereotactic cerebral atlasses were the roadmaps of functional neurosurgery in the era of ventriculography and arteriography, but the advent of modern neuroimaging techniques makes available highly detailed anatomical information of the cerebral parenchyma, obtained from individual patients, and anticipates the evolution of future "functional" atlasses. So far the development of CT and MRI techniques, and the introduction of localizing instruments for image acquisition under stereotactic conditions has opened a whole world of applications of stereotaxy in the field of visible target surgery, while functional procedures have been carried out only in a few Institutions, where the availability of anatomically detailed images has not replaced the traditional use of stereotactic atlasses. The superiority of ventriculography over CT in defining the classic intraventricular landmarks, and the unpredicatable distortion suffered from MRI images, may explain the reluctance to discard a well established procedure. This is a correct decision since it is virtually impossible to safely replace the use of a traditional atlas by digital images whose thickness, orientation, and in case of MRI, distortion, has many complications against questionable advantages. On the other hand cerebral atlasses will always be needed, not only to perform functional procedures, but also in the field of open surgery, where the perspective of extension of guided microsurgical procedures will sharpen the need for an atlas of cerebral functions, to superimpose on all available morphological data. In both cases, the atlas is going to lose its importance as an anatomical guide: histological information is probably of little importance, when compared to the statistical distribution of neurofunctional observations recorded in individual cases, when defining the most suitable target for functional procedures. The morphology of the model permits anatomical correspondence with the individual under scrunity, but the mathematical process involved will eventually identify a functional target, by showing how observations can be superimposed on the anatomy of a single case, following anatomical matching.

Material and Methods

A sequence of steps leads to the determination of the set of curvilinear coordinates for the best fit between an atlas and an individual case, and the solution to the problem of labelling neuroanatomical images. The main difficulty is dealing with individual variability in the use of a traditional atlas: simply matching planar sections of a model and of an individual brain is impossible because points of one section will find their corresponding points on a curved surface of the other brain. For this reason, solutions that take into account scale factors along the three axes[1,4,6] or modelling of structures according to polar coordinates[5] are unsatisfactory.

An ideal solution would be the introduction of standard anatomical coordinates in each brain by identification of homogeneous points in the two volumes and the consequential description of the curvilinear coordinate transformation. This 3-D matching solution has been developed to map one MRI acquisition of a patient over another, obtained from a different patient, with the same imaging method; For every point in volume A, a corresponding point is found in volume B that gives the best cross-correlative value of the signal contained in two 3-D windows moved around the points[3].

The lack of an ideal model atlas, consisting of a brain sectioned and stained after 3-D MRI acquisition, has prompted us to run a matching algorithm between a 3-D MRI acquisition and a traditional stereotactic atlas. The cross-correlative process can only function when the two data volumes contain the same kind of information, therefore the matching can be performed up to the available level of resolution between gray and white matter and CSF. Segmentation of MRI acquisitions needs to be performed in order to identify homogeneous regions to which a descriptive label is associated. Segmentation of MRI images requires a pre-processing phase to solve problems relating to the type of acquisition, among which the most relevant are, the non uniformity of gain within the

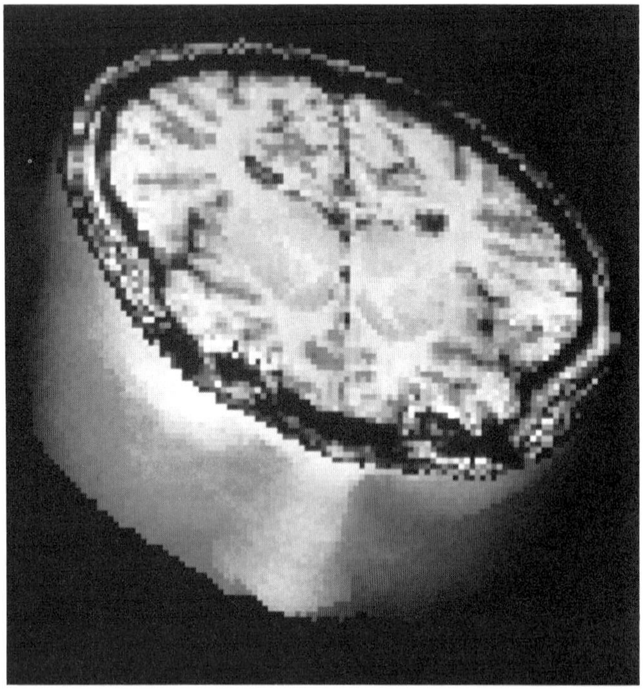

Fig. 1. The segmented volume of a "flash 3-D" MRI acquisition

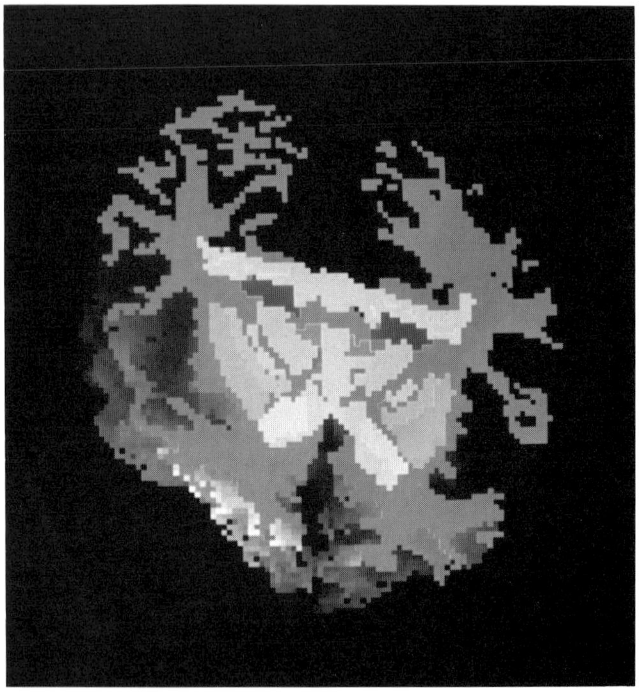

Fig. 2. A 3-D model atlas, whose morphological resolution is equivalent to the MRI segmented data.

image volume, noise and poor spatial resolution. Spatial resolution depends on acquisition time and is consequently related to the volume of data that can be reasonably processed. Noise can be reduced through statistical filtering of the volume, which reduces the signal scattering within homogeneous areas of the image[2]. The non-uniformity of gain can be adaptively compensated for by correction of the value of signal with a gain function, until the highest possible dynamic of the histogram is reached.

Discussion

This segmentation procedure can disclose geometrical information sufficiently detailed to automatically generate a copy of a neuroanatomical atlas, adapted to the patient's geometry (Figs. 1 and 2). Having solved the inaccuracy related to the different curvilinear coordinates, clinical and neurophysiological observations contained in the atlas can be transferred through the same coordinate transformation on the patient's geometry, with a geometric dispersion due only to topological differences or to the diffuse localization of some functions. Functional regions will have "fuzzy" limits, representing the probability of occurrence of observations.

References

1. Bertrand G, Olivier A (1974) Computer display of stereotaxic brain maps and probe tracks. Acta Neurochir (Wien) 21: 235–243
2. Borroni M, Turrin A *et al* (1985) Performance evaluation of some noise-smoothing techniques for Gamma camera digital images. Nucl Med Allied Sci 29: 245–251
3. Cerchiari U, Del Panno G *et al* (1987) 3-D correlation technique for anatomical volumes in functional stereotactic neurosurgery. In: Cappellini V (ed) Time-varying image processing and moving object recognition. Elsevier Science Publisher B.V. North Holland, pp 147–152
4. Hardy T, Koch J (1982) Computer assisted stereotactic surgery. Appl Neurophysiol 45: 396–398
5. Kall B A, Kelly P J (1985) Methodology and clinical experience with computed tomography and a computer resident stereotactic atlas. Neurosurgery 17: 400–406
6. Vries J K, McLinden S (1988) Computerized three-dimensional stereotactic atlasses. In: Lunsford L D (ed) Modern stereotactic neurosurgery. Martinus Nijhoff Publishing, Boston, pp 441–459

Correspondence: C. Giorgi, Department of Neurosurgery, Istituto Neurologico, Milano, Italy.

Brain Tumours, Stereotactical and Radiosurgical Management

Acta Neurochirurgica, Suppl. 52, 75–77 (1991)

The Stereotactic Approach to Brain Stem Lesions: A Follow-up of 29 Cases

S. Blond[1], **J.P. Lejeune, T. Dupard, M. Parent, J. Clarisse,** and **J.L. Christiaens**

[1]Department of Neurosurgery, C.H.R.U., Lille, France

Summary

Stereotactic biopsy is the safest and most reliable method for the histological diagnosis of intraaxial brain stem lesions. The definitive pathological diagnosis permits the selection of adequate therapy. No operative and/or adjuvant therapy must be proposed without a previous histological diagnosis. This approach avoids the complication of inappropriate therapy and provides valuable prognostic information.

Keywords: Brain stem lesions; stereotactical biopsy; management.

Introduction

The diagnosis and management of brain lesions are made easier with the information of modern imaging (C.T. and/or M.R.I.): these neuroradiological explorations provide an accurate and reliable location of these lesions but not the pathological diagnosis. A well-adapted therapeutic strategy of intracranial mass lesions is only possible after the exact knowledge of the histological characteristics. A tumour with exophytic component in the fourth ventricle or in the cisterns may be easily approached and even subtotally removed, but when the lesion is diffuse and intrinsic, we know that open biopsy procedures represent a major invasive surgical operation and frequently provide negative or inadequate sampling of the lesion. In these cases, the therapy has often been empirical in spite of the great heterogeneity of the brain stem lesions.

Epstein[5] has even written that "there is no useful information to be obtained from biopsy and that the overwhelming majority of brain stem neoplasms are malignant". With the widespread implementation of stereotactic techniques in neurosurgery, we may prove the extreme polymorphism of brain stem lesions and do not support that opinion. The use of the Talairach's system guided by C.T. or M.R.I. allows a safe and reliable approach to this vital area by a frontal or a suboccipital transcerebellar trajectory according to the site of the lesion. In some rare cases, this procedure may be the basis of linear accelerator-based radiosurgery.

Material and Methods

From January 1985 to July 1990, from a total of 360 stereotactic biopsy procedures, 29 patients with space occupying lesions of the brain stem underwent this procedure. 12 patients were children, 17 adults. Twelve were female and seventeen male with an age range from 7 to 68 years (m = 27.8). The preoperative symptomatic period extended from 4 weeks to 7 years and included cranial nerve symptoms and slight motor deficit. In seven cases, there was an occlusive hydrocephalus requiring ventriculo-peritoneal shunt. All patients underwent high resolution C.T. with thin and continuous slices, with and without contrast infusion. The more recent cases had preoperative M.R.I. (three planes in T1 weighted; sagittal plane in T2 weighted: systematic injection of gadolinium in T1). For the late cases these explorations have been completed by a three-dimensional computerized definition of the target and calculation of the angle of the probe trajectory.

The stereotactic exploration was performed under general anaesthesia: the Talairach frame was placed in low position and we used the Sceratti instrument for the double obliquity approach. In every cases, angiography and ventriculography were performed to visualize the relationship of the lesion to vessels (basilar, posterior cerebral and vertebral arteries; internal cerebral veins) and aqueduct of Sylvius. After manual or computerized transposition of data from C.T. scan and/or M.R.I., a target, if possible including an area with contrast enhancement, was chosen. Twenty-eight patients with lesions in or near the midline of the brain stem underwent operation using a transfrontal approach: the entry point was at the coronal suture; the probe trajectory traverses the lateral ventricle and the caudal diencephalon and midbrain. In one case with a lesion of the middle cerebellar peduncle, the approach was suboccipital transcerebellar. In 11 cases, the biopsy was proceeded by electrical monopolar stimulation (5 to 50 Hz with 1 ms pulse width, up to 1OV) to minimize the risk of encroaching upon motor pathways. Generally, two to three samples are taken with the Sedan-Vallicioni instrument. Small fragments are taken at both ends of the sample for hematoxylin-eosin stained smear preparations. Intraoperative histological diagnosis gives valuable cytologic information. The final histologic diagnosis is based on glutaraldehyde fixed paraffin embedded material, available usually in 48 hours. Several histological features are examined: nature, grading and, if possible, the spatial configuration.

Results

The location of the brain stem lesions was in the diencephalon-mesencephalon in 10 cases, in the mesencephalon in 10 cases, in the pons in 6 cases and in the medulla in three cases. Pathological diagnoses were obtained in all patients. The results of biopsies are listed in the Table 1. The data illustrate the extreme polymorphism of the histological diagnoses: one primary peduncular haematoma with cryptic telangiectasia, two metastases which were the first signs of occult malignancy, one toxoplasmosis (associated with AIDS). There were two cases of gliosis. Gliomas, whatever the location, of all grades could be present in all the different locations.

In two cases, the post-operative period was marked by a transient aggravation of a preexisting neurological deficit but no intracerebral haemorrhage could be demonstrated with C.T. scan.

Table 1. *Histological Results*

	Results	
Location	Nature	Grading
Diencephalon Mesencephalon: 10	– 3 Oligodendroglioma	II, III, I
	– 3 Astrocytoma	III
	– 1 Pilocytic Astrocytoma	
	– 1 Centroblastic Lymphoma	
	– 1 Naevocarcinoma	
	– 1 Metastasis	
Mesencephalon: 10	– 2 Gliosis	
	– 3 Oligodendrocytoma	I, II, III
	– 2 Astrocytoma	I, III
	– 1 Teratoma	
	– 1 Toxoplasmosis	
	– 1 Pinealocytoma	
Pons : 6	– 1 Haematoma (Telangectasia)	
	– 1 Oligoastrocytoma	III
	– 3 Astrocytoma	II, III, III
	– 1 Metastasis	
Medulla : 3	– 1 Oligodendroglioma	I
	– 1 Oligoastrocytoma	II
	– 1 Astrocytoma	III

Discussion

C.T. and M.R.I. provide excellent information about the precise location of brain stem lesions and their relation to adjacent structures. However, no histological conclusion is possible. Without this diagnosis, there is a great risk of inappropriate and/or empirical therapy. Until later years, brain stem biopsies were considered too dangerous, and irradiation without histological verification was carried out with the tentative diagnosis of a brain stem glioma. No doubt, an intrinsic brain stem lesion can be stereotactically biopsied with low morbidity and no mortality.

In view of our results from this series, we cannot support the opinion of Matson: "Exploration for histological confirmation of brain stem tumours should be avoided because the outcome was always poor".[8] Our experience is similar to that of Broggi[2], Coffey and Lunsford[3–4], and Guthrie[6] who have proven the accuracy and the safety of stereotactic biopsies with different systems: Riechert, Leksell, Brown-Robert-Wells. The usefulness of integrating imaging techniques with a stereotactic approach is evident since it makes high precision biopsies possible. The safety of the Talairach's methodology, already demonstrated by Munari[9], is due to a precise recognition of the topographical relationship between the lesion and neighbouring cerebral structures with important functional properties. The transfrontal approach permits a trajectory to all divisions of the brain stem. When the lesion is more lateral, in the pons or in the middle cerebellar peduncle, the most direct route is the suboccipital-transcerebellar.

The analysis of the histological results demonstrates the extreme heterogeneity of glial brain stem tumours with variable degrees of histologic malignancy. It is essential to perform, if possible, multiple biopsies to enable a complete histopathological diagnosis which is a prerequisite for adequate treatment. In two cases, the diagnoses have been non-neoplasic lesions: aspiration of an old peduncular haemorrhage with presence of telangiectasia; toxoplasmosis leading to the diagnosis of acquired immune-deficiency syndrome. Among the neoplasic lesions, biopsies revealed a primary centroblastic lymphoma and a neurocarcinoma. In another case, the diagnosis of a radioresistent lesion (teratoma) made ineffective, external irradiation unnecessary. These date indicate that radiation therapy should not be carried out for brain stem intrinsic lesions without an histological diagnosis.

References

1. Betti O, Dereckinski V (1983) Irradiation stereotaxique multi-faisceaux. Neurochirurgie 29: 295–298
2. Broggi G, Franzini A, Giorgi C (1983) The value of stereotactic biopsy in management of brain-stem lesions. Slow growing cerebral tumours. Ital J Neurol Sci [Suppl] 2: 51–56
3. Coffey RJ, Lunsford LD, (1985) Stereotactic surgery for mass lesions of the midbrain and pons. Neurosurgery 17: 12–17
4. Coffey RJ, Lunsford LD (1985) Diagnosis and treatment of brain stem mass lesions by CT guided stereotactic surgery. Appl Neurophysiol 48: 467–471
5. Epstein F(1985) A staging system for brain stem gliomas. Cancer 56: 1804–1806
6. Guthrie BL, Steinberg GK, Adler JR (1989) Posterior foss a stereotaxic biopsy using the Brown-Roberts Wells stereotaxis system. J Neurosurg 70: 649–652
7. Hood TW, Gebarski SS, McKeever PE, Venes JL (1986) Stereotaxis biopsy of intrinsic lesions of the brain stem. J Neurosurg 65: 172–176
8. Matson DD (1969) Neurosurgery of infancy and childhood, Ed. 2, Springfied, Charles C, Thomas, pp 469–477
9. Munari C, Musolino A, Rosler JR, Blond S, Demierre B, Betti O, Daumas-Duport C, Missir O, Chodkiewics JP (1987) Stereotactic approach to space occupying lesion in the posterior fossa. Appl Neurophysiol 50: 200–202

Correspondence: S. Blond, Department of Neurosurgery, C.H.R.U., F-59037 Lille, France.

Acta Neurochirurgica, Suppl. 52, 78–80 (1991)

A New Surgical but less Invasive Treatment of Central Brain Tumours Preliminary Report

P.W. Ascher, E. Justich[1], und O. Schröttner

Universitätskliniken für Neurochirurgie and [1]Radiologie, Graz, Austria

Summary

Our goal was always to reduce the risks of anaesthesia and surgery to a minimum. Therefore we introduced the interstitial thermotherapy of central brain tumours. The center of the tumour is calculated with the help of computer tomography, then we reach the target stereotactically. The last step includes the insertion of a Nd:YAG laser fiber and the denaturation of the tumour under real time magnetic resonance control. The whole procedure is carried out in local anaesthesia. Methods and first clinical results are demonstrated.

Keywords: Central brain tumours; stereotactic thermotherapy; ND:YAG laser – tumour denaturation; real time MR control.

Introduction

Tumours of the brain can kill the patient not only by malignancy but also by invading central, surgically in accessable structures, which may apply also to beinign tumours. Some of these tumours, long considered inoperable, have been treated by interstitial brachytherapy.

In 1984 an eight year old boy presented at our department with left-sided hemiplegia. A computed tomography (CT) scan showed a tumour in the right posterior thalamus. A biopsy of the tumour was obtained by sterotactic needle puncture and a newly designed endoscope. Histology showed an astrocytoma, grade II. Because the tumour was inoperable according to conventional standards, a $1.06\,\mu$ Nd:YAG laser was used to irradiate the portion of the tumour visibly protruding into the posterior horn of the lateral ventricle. A dose of 50,000 Joule (enough to bring a cup of water to boil) was applied to the surface of the tumour during continuous cooling by irrigation with saline. The surface of the tumour, previously pink, paled visibly during the procedure. Hemiplegia resolved within a week. CT scans 2 months and 4 years after surgery showed no evidence of residual tumour.

A 35 year old female with a similar tumour was treated the same way a few months later[1,2]. This therapeutic approach seems appropriate only for paraventricular tumours of the thalamus which are rare.

A potential disadvantage of the procedure is the high power density at the end of the laser fiber which damages the fiber tip. A further problem is intraoperative temperature control of the radiated tissue.

Two developments occurred in 1986: 1. Contact laser tips became available, 2. G. Jako and F. Jolesch[3] demonstrated that the heat effect of laser fibers in the brain could be monitored continuously in nearly real time (3 minutes delay) by magnetic resonance (MR) imaging.

Clinical studies showed that the heat effect of laser irradiation was visible two hours later. In the meantime the company MBB-AT has designed a completely new fiber system that has proven effective in experiments and clinical practice.

In vitro experiments on porcine liver at room temperature showed that 4 Watts applied over 10 minutes caused an ellipsoid coagulation necrosis of 12-16 mm. Two fibers simultaneously heated do not cause a double volume necrosis but a new geometry and much bigger necrosis. The calibration of the laser source (MBB 50 Watts laser) was stable during all experiments.

Indications

All benign or malignant central brain tumours in patients without neurologic symptoms are indications for interstitial thermotherapy (ITT). ITT has a number of advantages as compared with interstitial brachytherapy. ITT is a simple procedure, the heat reaction of the tumour and surrounding tissue can be monitored directly and ITT can be performed on all types of tumours. ITT also has the advantages associated with brachytherapy: only local anaesthesia is required, sensomotoric function and speech can be evaluated continuously, the procedure can be repeated and the stereotactic approach permits minimal damage to the surrounding brain tissue[4].

Methods

On the morning of surgery a specially designed, plastic ring is placed on the patient's skull. The co-ordinates of the center of the tumour and those for an appropriate burrhole are plotted by CT. Trepanation is then carried out under local anesthesia. At the same time the co-ordinates of the target point and the burrhole are plotted on a phantom. An aiming device is adapted and then transferred to the co-ordinate ring on the patient's head, the probe is then implanted. Afterwards the patient is taken to the MR unit and the laser fiber is introduced to the calculated length under MR control (Fig. 1).

The laser is then activated (4 Watts, 10 minutes). The first changes in the tumour become apparent on the MR screen after 5 minutes. Further laser applications are adapted according to the size of the lesion and the observed heat reaction (Fig 2, a,b,c). The patient is monitored physiologically during the entire procedure. None of the 8 patients to date have reported pain or other sensations. The greatest difficulty is the 10 minutes' motionless fixation of the patient.

Most of our instruments are now MR compatible. Only the aiming device and the fixation of the probe remain to be redesigned.

Discussion

ITT permits treatment for otherwise untreatable brain tumours without endangering patients function

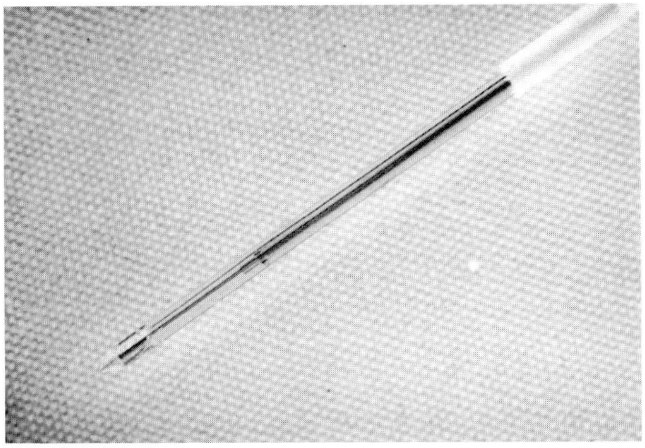

Fig. 1. Laser fiber for interstitial thermotherapy with an air chamber at the end of the fiber

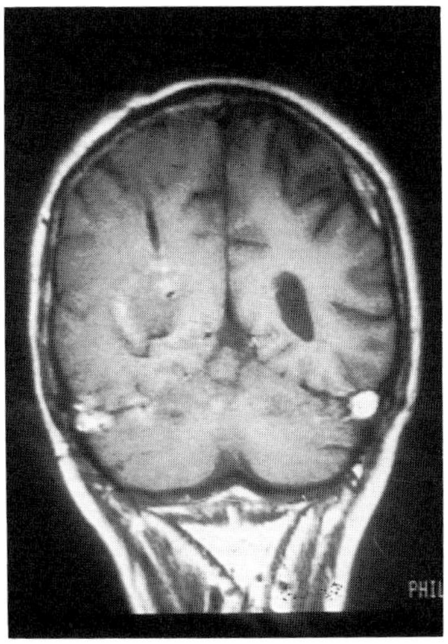

a

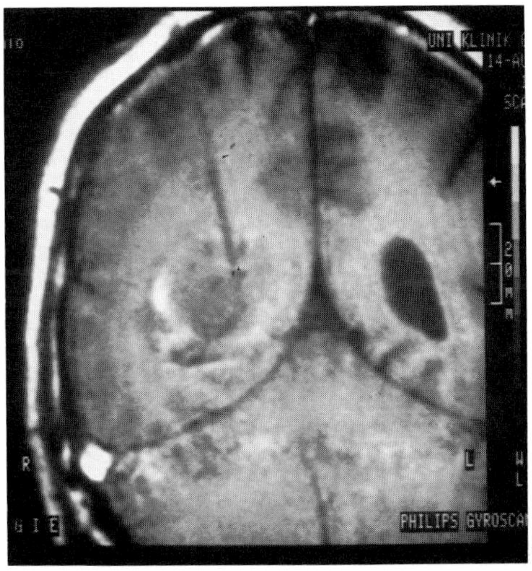

b

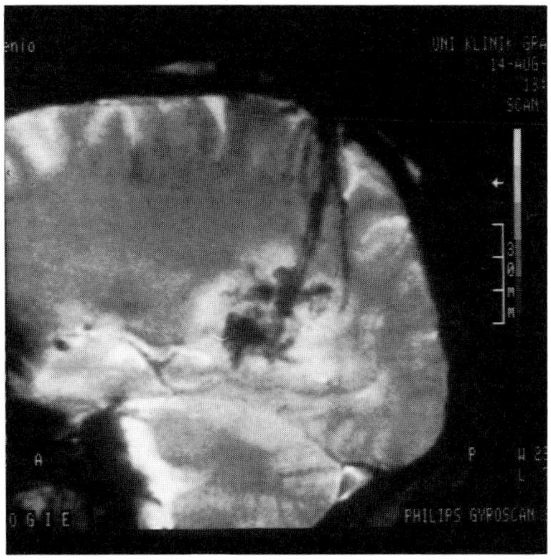

c

Fig. 2. (a) MR control with probe implanted in the tumour before denaturation (T_1), (b) the same patient after 3 minutes of coagulation (T_1), (c) the tumour after denaturation, 10 minutes radiation time

or life. ITT is a palliative measure for malignant tumours, for benign lesions it may offer cure.

A number of technical problems (equipment, both instrumentation and MR), experiments (heat distribution) and clinical studies (histology, long term follow-up) remain to be done and solved, but ITT has opened a new vista in the treatment of central brain tumours.

Correspondence: P.W. Ascher, Universitätskliniken für Neurochirurgie, Karl-Franzens Universität Graz, A-8036 Graz, Austria.

Acta Neurochirurgica, Suppl. 52, 81–83 (1991)

Stereotactic Laser Therapy in Cerebral Gliomas

M. Bettag[1], **F. Ulrich**[1], **R. Schober**[2], **G. Fürst**[3], **K.J. Langen**[4], **M. Sabel**[1], and **J.C.W. Kiwit**[1]

Departments of [1]Neurosurgery, [2] Neuropathology, [3] Diagnostic Radiology and [4] Nuclear Medicine, Heinrich-Heine-University Dusseldorf, Germany

Summary

The 1.06 μm Nd:YAG laser and a new fiberoptic delivery system, the Interstitial Thermo-Therapy (ITT) laser fibre, allows stereotactic interstitial irradiation of cerebral tumours. In experimental rat brain studies we found typical laser-tissue effects with a central necrosis and a sharply demarcated oedema towards the normal brain. The size of the lesion depended on the energy and exposure time applied.

In a pilot series we treated 5 patients with cerebral gliomas WHO grade II-III in functionally important regions and monitored the therapeutic effects by MR imaging and PET scan. Early post-operative results showed irreversible necrotic changes in the tumour centre and reversible oedematous changes at the tumour margin. Long-term results will show if stereotactic interstitial laser therapy is a useful supplementary method in the treatment of malignant cerebral tumours.

Keywords: Cerebral gliomas; lasers; local hyperthermia.

Introduction

Hyperthermia is an accepted method in the treatment of malignant tumours. The 1.06 μm Nd: YAG laser and its new fiberoptic delivery system, the Interstitial Thermo-Therapy (ITT) laser fibre, is an excellent source of local hyperthermia and allows interstitial irradiation of cerebral tumours.

Material and Methods

Laser-induced Interstitial Thermo-Therapy was performed by use of a Nd:YAG laser with a wavelength of 1.06 μm and the ITT laser fibre. It was applied in an experimental model on normal rat brains. The ITT laser fibre with an outer diameter of 1.2 mm was introduced stereotactically (David Kopf Instruments stereotactic system) through a right frontal burrhole. Laser shots were emitted as continuous waves with an output power of 2–5 watts in a single focus. The exposure time ranged from 30 sec. to 5 min. For histological examination rat brains were removed immediately, 1 day, 3 days, 1 week and 2 weeks following laser therapy.

In a first clinical trial, 5 patients with gliomas WHO grade II-III were treated by stereotactic interstitial laser therapy. Two gliomas were located in the central motor cortex, one in the thalamus and two in the medio-basal temporal lobe. The size of the tumours ranged from 1 to 3.5 cm in diameter. Therapeutic effects were controlled by contrast enhanced CT scan, Gd-DTPA enhanced MR imaging and PET scan using FDG. All CT and MR and two PET studies were performed preoperatively, 1–3 days and 7–9 days after laser therapy.

Results

Histological examination of rat brains removed immediately after laser therapy revealed typical laser effects. The size of the lesion depended on the power and the exposure time. We found a central coagulative necrosis with a sharply demarcated peripheral oedema. Laser irradiation using laser parameters of 2–4 watts over a period of 30–120 sec. resulted in small circumscribed lesions of 3–5 mm in diameter. Application of 4–5 watts with an exposure time of 4–5 min. affected nearly a whole hemisphere. However, the histological features were always the same. Histological examination of rat brains removed 1–2 weeks after laser therapy showed central defects and coagulative necroses surrounded by resorptive changes with a small oedematous rim.

In our clinical study, we observed specific laser-tissue changes in CT scan and MR imaging in 3 of 5 patients with cerebral gliomas. Early postoperative Gd-DTPA enhanced MR images obtained 24–36 hours after laser therapy showed a marked decrease of enhancement in the centre of the glioma and a small annular, highly increased uptake at the tumour margin (Figs. 1 and 2). One week later, MRI revealed an increase of the size of the lesion (Fig. 3). PET studies using FDG confirmed these results. One day after laser therapy there was a loss of glucose uptake in the

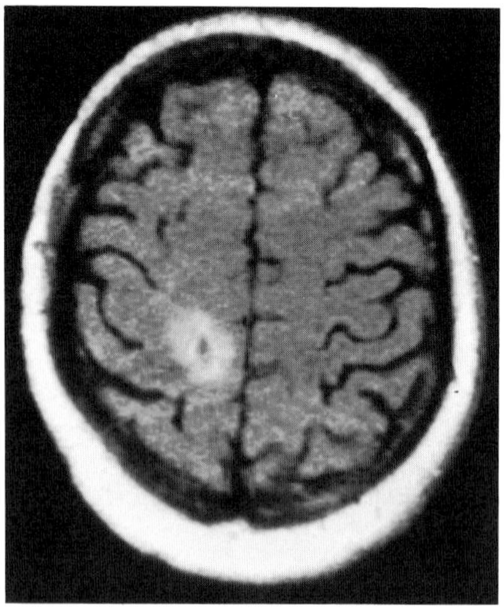

Fig. 1. Pretherapeutic post-Gd-DTPA T_1weighted SE (500/30) images demonstrate a homogeneous enhancement of an astrocytoma WHO grade II-III. The dot inside the tumour is due to a lesion after prior diagnostic stereotactic biopsy

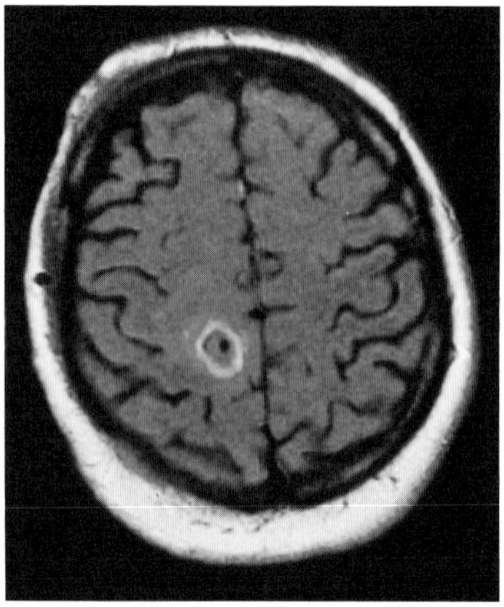

Fig. 2. 24 hours after laser therapy using 4 watts over a period of 5 min. in two foci, a marked decrease of Gd accumulation in the centre of the tumour is seen. Ring-shaped increased enhancement at the tumour margin

tumour centre and a hypermetabolic rim at the tumour margin. One week later, the lesion has become larger in size with glucose uptake at the tumour margin now being in normal range.

Discussion

Heat has been used to treat tumours for at least 100 years by various invasive and noninvasive techniques[2]. There is also the possibility to use lasers for inducing

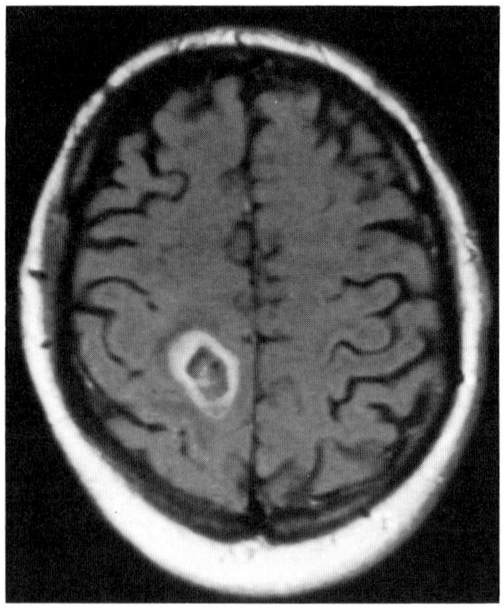

Fig. 3. One week later MR image shows laser-tissue effects being larger in size

hyperthermia in malignancies[6]. The advantage of lasers is the very precise delivery of energy to tissue and the good instrumental control of total energy deposition[3]. Particularly the Nd:YAG laser with its wavelength of 1.06 μm and its new fiberoptic system, the ITT laser fibre, is an excellent tool for interstitial laser therapy of cerebral tumours. Thermal effects are maximized by use of low power densities and long exposure times[8].

Until now, specific laser effects on brain tissue were mainly analysed by histological studies and measurements of temperature distribution[5]. We used MR imaging and PET scan as noninvasive and sensitive methods of visualizing the qualitative and spatial extent of laser-tissue interactions in cerebral gliomas. Laser irradiation induces changes not only in the thermal motions of the hydrogen photons but also in the distribution and mobility of water and lipids[1]. These alterations result in changed relaxation times. The strong temperature dependance of MR relaxation has been shown in several investigations[1,7]. The main changes in tissue parameters seem to occur in T_1-weighted images. In our studies, MRI and PET scan revealed irreversible necrotic changes in the tumour centre after laser therapy. At the tumour margin we found transitory oedematous changes. The fact that tissue effects became larger in size after one week may indicate that laser-tissue interactions do not only appear at the time of application but progress with a certain period. However, improved control of exact volumetric determination of laser energy deposition may be possible by using real time high speed MR sequences so that imaging can keep pace with the time-scale of laser-induced thermal changes[4].

References

1. Bottomley PA, Foster TH, Argersinger RE, Pfeifer LM (1984) A review of normal tissue hydrogen NMR relaxation times and relaxation mechanisms from 1–100 MHz: Dependency on tissue type, NMR frequency, temperature, species, excision, and age. Med Phys 11: 42–448
2. Busch W (1866) Über den Einfluß welchen heftigere Erysipeln zuweilen auf organisierte Neubildungen ausüben. Verhandl Naturh Preuss Rhein, Westphal 23: 28–30
3. Cummins L, Nauenberg M (1983) Thermal effects of laser radiation in biological tissue. Biophys J 42: 90–102
4. Jolesz FA, Bleier AR, Jakab P, Ruenzel PW, Huttl K, Jako GJ (1988) MR imaging of laser-tissue interactions. Radiology 168: 249–253
5. Lajat Y, Patrice T, Nomballais F, Nogues B, Resche F (1987) Effects of 1.06 μm wavelength laser radiation applied stereotactically to brain tissue. Laser Surg Med 3: 45–51
6. Mang TS, Dougherty TJ (1986) Use of the Nd: YAG laser for hyperthermia induction as an adjunct to photodynamic therapy. Laser Surg Med 6: 237
7. Parker DL, Smith V, Sheldon P, Crooks LE, Fussel L (1983) Temperature distribution measurements in two-dimensional NMR imaging. Med Phys 10: 321–325
8. Welch AJ (1984) The thermal response of laser irradiated tissue. IEEE J Quantum Electronics 20: 1471–1481

Correspondence: M. Bettag, Neurochirurgische Klinik der Heinrich-Heine-Universität Düsseldorf, Moorenstr. 5, D-W-4000 Düsseldorf 1, Federal Republic of Germany.

Acta Neurochirurgica, Suppl. 52, 84–86 (1991)

Development of a Second Generation Stereotactic Apparatus for Linear Accelerator Radiosurgery

F. Colombo*, L. Casentini[1], F. Pozza[2], G. Chierego[3], and C. Marchetti[3]

Departments of [1]Neurosurgery, [2]Radiotherapy and [3]Medical Physics, City Hospital, Vicenza, Italy

Summary

Linear accelerator radiosurgery technique is based on a multiple intersecting arc irradiations procedure. The coincidence of the axis of two rotation movements (of gantry and treatment couch) into the isocenter is critical for focusing irradiation.

In October 1989, our linear accelerator was changed and the stereotactic apparatus had to be adapted to the new machine. After multiple mechanical tests of the new machine, the stereotactic head frame was fixed to the roller bearing allowing rotation of the couch. The new apparatus is described.

Keywords: Focal irradiation; Linear accelerator; stereotactic apparatus.

Introduction

In our department, from 1982 to 1989, we employed an original linear accelerator radiosurgical technique based on multiple intersecting arc irradiations, focused on the stereotactic target[1]. The target was fixed by a special stereotactic frame to the treatment couch of the linear accelerator (linac) and was made to coincide with the isocentre by controlled movements of the treatment couch. Arc irradiations were performed in different planes obtained by the rotation of the treatment couch-stereotactic apparatus assembled around a vertical axis passing through the isocenter. The accuracy with which the target is hit by the moving beam depends on the mechanical characteristics of the linac: that is, the coincidence with the isocenter of both gantry and couch axis of rotation. Moreover, if the stereotactic frame is fixed to the treatment couch, the latter must be sufficiently steady to maintain coincidence of the target with the isocenter during rotation movements. This geometrical accuracy, as a general characteristic of linacs, has always been challenged by supporters of static, multiple cobalt sources, radiosurgical units. In October 1989, owing to mechanical wear, we had to replace the linear accelerator and a Siemes Mevatron 6 MV was selected for upgrading our radiosurgical unit. A new stereotactic apparatus had to be developed to comply with the new machine and to meet particular needs of technical refinements that came out after the introduction of the first generation stereotactic device.

Material and Methods

This apparatus has to comply with four main requirements:

1) The apparatus must guarantee the mechanical accuracy needed for precise irradiation of targets in the range of 3 to 4 mm (with our smallest collimator of 5 mm).

2) Head frame and its support must not interfere with the rotation of the radiation source.

3) Head frame and its support must be easily removable for allowing beside radiosurgery and standard radiotherapy activity.

4) The system must allow radiosurgical treatment of 3-D irregular targets, following an original procedure, based on controlled rectilinear movements of the target during irradiation[2].

The new linear accelerator underwent a complete series of mechanical tests. The accuracy of the rotation of the gantry around the isocenter is around 0.6 mm. This accuracy is completely dependent on the manufacturer, that has to comply with accepted standards. On the other hand, flexion entailed by different loads (up to 80 kg) shifted the cranial extremity of the couch by 4 mm. A lateral thrust of 30 kg applied to the top of the table moved the extremity 8 mm controlaterally.

In order to correct this mechanical deficiency, the body of the couch was dismantled and the point of maximal flexion was found to be the plate connecting the couch to the roller bearing embedded in the concrete of the floor. One other source of possible misalignment under strain was found in the torsion of the support of the table. The main roller bearing proved to be unaffected by the load (less than 0.05 mm movement for 80 kg on the couch, no

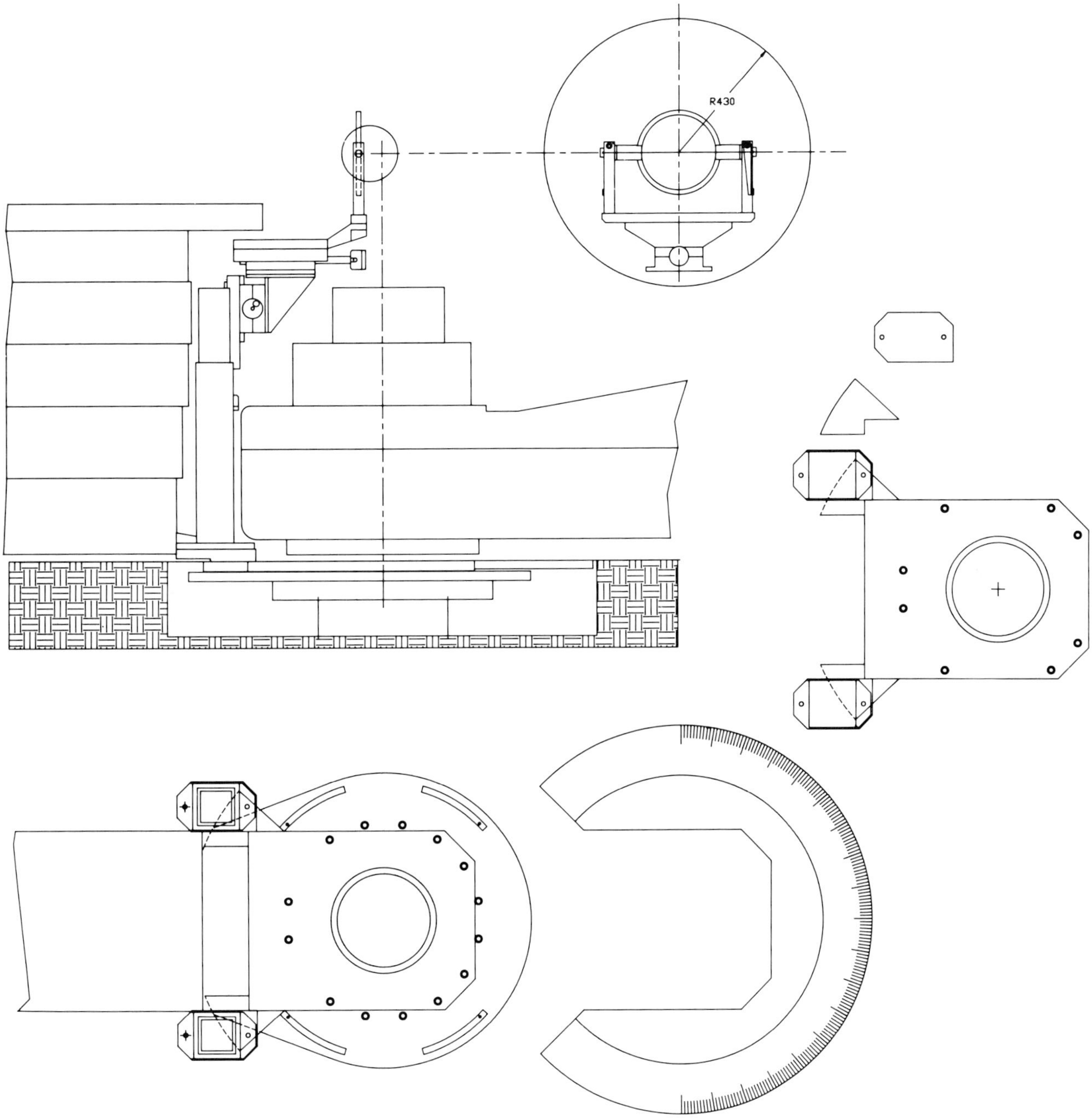

Fig. 1. Technical drawing of stereotactic apparatus

influence of lateral thrust) and was selected as the base for the support of the new stereotactic apparatus.

Results

The second generation stereotactic apparatus (Figs. 1, 2) comprises two rigid steel pillars to which three orthogonal slides are bolted. The base ring is fixed to the slides by an adaptor. The entire apparatus can be easily removed and precisely repositioned by a specially designed crane. The base ring is moved according to the tree coordinates to make the target coincide with the isocenter. These movements can be operated by computer controlled motors, thus allowing 3-D radiosurgery. Flexion induced by load are less than 0.4 mm in the worst conditions (30 kg, lateral thrust), below the limit of tolerance of high precision radiosurgical treatment. After a complete dosimetric vertification on anthropomorphic and

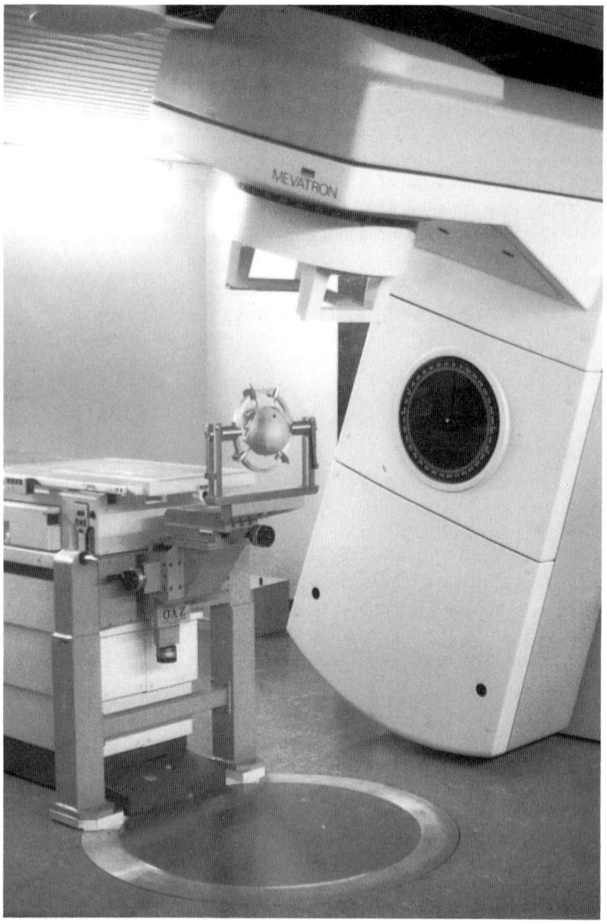

Fig. 2. The apparatus is fixed to the linear accelerator

polyethylene phantoms, the apparatus has been used in clinical practice.

Discussion

Radiosurgical practice should be able to deal with very small intracranial targets (for example, arterial feeders of an arteriovenous malformation)[3]. Without a thorough mechanical and physical evaluation, linear accelerator radiosurgery runs the risk of missing the target. Different linear accelerators require dedicated stereotactic frames designed for minimizing mechanical error. The need for close cooperation between the radiosurgery team and the linear accelerator manufacturer is emphasized.

References

1. Colombo F, Benedetti A, Pozza F, Avanzo RC, Chierego G, Marchetti C (1985) Stereotactic external irradiation by linear accelerator. Neurosurgery 16: 154–160
2. Colombo F, Benedetti A, Zanardo A, Pozza F, Avanzo R, Chierego G, Marchetti C (1987) New technique for three-dimensional linear accelerator radiosurgery. Acta Neurochir (Wien) [Suppl] 39: 38–40
3. Steiner L, Leksell L, Forster DMC, Greitz T, Backlund EO (1974) Stereotactic radiosurgery in intracranial arteriovenous malformations. Acta Neurochir (Wien) [Suppl] 21: 195–209

Correspondence: F. Colombo, Department of Neurosurgery, City Hospital, Viale Rodolfi 37, I-36100 Vicenza, Italy.

Acta Neurochirurgica, Suppl. 52, 87–89 (1991)

Gamma Knife Surgery for Cerebral Metastasis

L. Kihlström, B. Karlsson, Ch. Lindquist, G. Norén, and **T. Rähn**

Department of Neurosurgery, Karolinska Institute, Stockholm, Sweden

Summary

Twentysix cerebral metastatic tumours treated with the Gamma knife employing a large single dose were followed by repeated clinical and CT examinations. In most cases Gamma knife surgery was the only treatment. The follow up time has been longer than 6 months with a median follow up of 9 months. In all but one of the cases a remarkable progressive shrinkage of the tumour started 2–4 months after the therapy. The therapeutic results indicate that radiosurgery used even as the only form of treatment is the best treatment alternative for cerebral metastasis presently available.

Keywords: Cerebral metastasis; radiosurgery; gamma knife surgery.

Introduction

It is estimated that cerebral metastasis occur in 20–40% of patients with systemic cancer[1]. Presently, surgical removal followed by whole brain radiotherapy (WBRT) offers the best treatment results[5,6]. In a recent prospective randomized study it was found that this combined therapy was accompanied by local recurrence of the metastasis in 20% of cases whereas radiotherapy alone was accompanied by a 50% recurrency rate[9]. However, surgery is in general considered a realistic alternative only with single metastatic tumours in patients in a good condition and with an expected survival time of more than 2 months[9].

Radiosurgery offers the possibility of delivering a very high dose of radiation in a single session, effectively restricted to the pathology to be treated and it has been shown that growth of metastatic tumours can be arrested by such a method[8]. It could thus be anticipated that Gamma Knife surgery would give treatment results comparable to those of surgery and WBRT in combination and with the additional important advantage of limiting the hospitalization to 1 day. These expectations were fulfilled in the treatment of a patient with a recurrent hypernephroma metastasis[3] and encouraged the continuation of the treatment policy the results of which are reported here.

Material and Methods

From 1975 to September of 1990, 44 patients with metastasis to the brain have been treated by radiosurgery in the Gamma Knife at our institution (Table 1). Twentysix tumours have been followed clinically and by CT for more than 6 months and form the basis of this report. During the period 1975 to March of 1988 the second prototype of the Gamma Knife was used. The configuration of this machine and the treatment techniques used with it have been previously described[4,7]. From 1988 a production model of the Gamma Knife has been used. The dose rate was 0.7–3 Gy/min in the prototype model and around 4 Gy/min in the newer model.

The tumours were localized by stereotactic CT-scan using intravenous contrast and the tumour volume was estimated. Smaller spherical tumours were then treated using a single volume of radiation with the 14 or 18 mm collimator. Larger tumours were treated with multiple isocenters. The median average dose was 53 Gy and the median minimum dose to the tumour was 31 Gy. The whole procedure was performed in local anaesthesia as a single session outpatient procedure. The pretreatment volumes of the metastases varied between 0.3 and 13 cm^3 with a median volume of 4.4 cm^3. Tumour volume assessments were also made on the follow-up CT-scans. These were planned for 3, 6 and 12 months after treatment and then annually.

Results

With these large single doses there was no difference in response between the tumours related to histology. In all cases but one there was a striking shrinkage of the tumours starting 2–4 months after the treatment. Three metastases from adenocarcinomas and 2 from melanomas disappeared completely 2 months – 1 year following treatment. Four of these tumours had a volume of 1 cm^3 or less and 1 had a pretreatment volume of 5 cm^3. Nineteen tumours in the volume

Table 1. *Cerebral Metastasis Primary Tumour Sites*

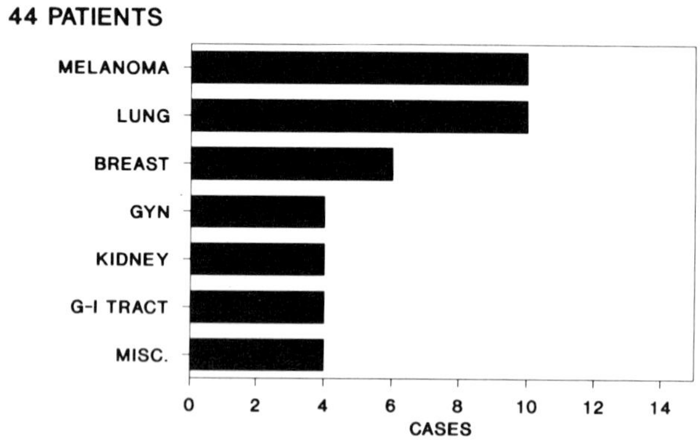

range 2–13 cm^3 decreased by 75% over a 3–6 months observation period. The only non-responder had a metastasis to the brainstem from an ovarian carcinoma and received only 13 Gy as the minimum dose to the tumour. This particular tumour increased in volume from 4 cm^3 to 7 cm^3 in 3 weeks from the time of diagnosis to the time of Gamma Knife surgery. Three months after treatment the volume had decreased by 50% but during the subsequent 3 months the volume again increased and neurological symptoms developed. Autopsy performed after her demise in bronchopneumonia 1 month later showed tumour cells and necrosis. With the exception of this case there were no cases in which neurological symptoms or signs progressed after radiosurgery and there were no "neurological deaths".

Case Reports

Case #1: A 50 year old man with angina pectoris and malignant melanoma treated by surgery the year before developing epileptic seizures. A CT-scan revealed a 1 cm^3 metastatic tumour (Fig. 1 a) which was treated by Gamma Knife surgery. The minimum dose was 50 Gy and the average dose 66 Gy. Six years later, there was no clinical indication of a recurrence and only a tissue scar was visible on the CT and MRI scans. (Figs. 1 b and c).

Case #2: A 75 year old man with 3 previous myocardial infarctions developed vertigo and ataxia from a gastrointestinal adenocarcinoma metastasis to the cerebellum. The tumour volume was 5 cm^3 and it was treated by an average dose of 71 Gy and a minimal dose of 25 Gy. After 3 months no tumour was visible on CT-scan and his cerebellar symptoms had decreased. To date, 1 year later, there has not been a recurrence. (Figs 2 a and b).

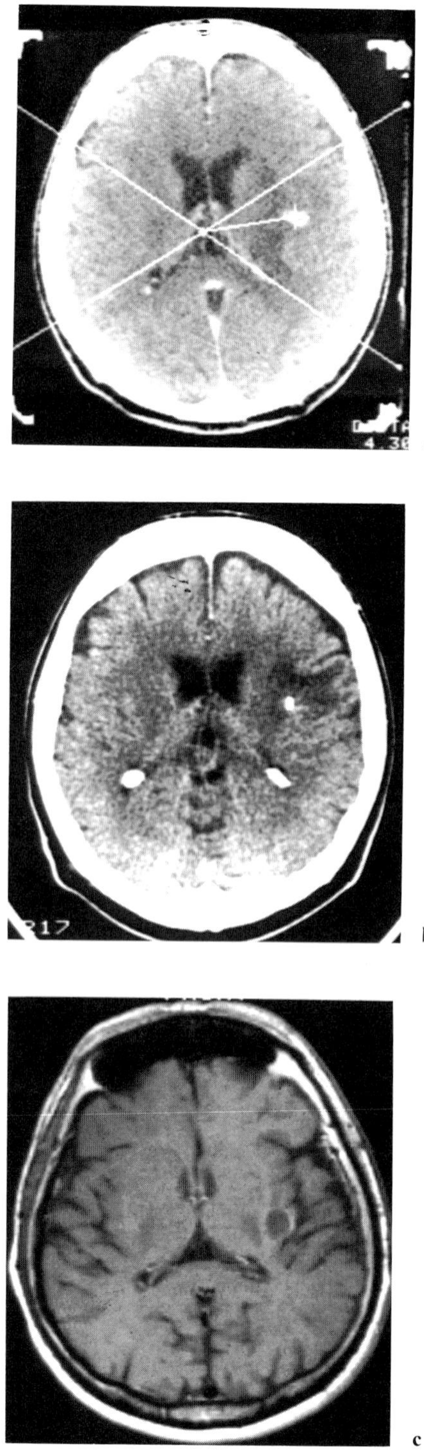

Fig. 1. Transaxial contrast-enhanced CT scans (a and b) and a T1W Gd-enhanced MRI scan (c) obtained in case #1 at Gamma Knife surgery (a), 3 (b) and 6 years (c) later

Discussion

Metastatic tumours of the central nervous system are manifestations of advanced cancers. The results of the treatment of the brain metastases heavily influence the length of survival with a median survival of only 1 month if left untreated[9]. The best currently available therapy, surgery in combination with WBRT, has several disadvantages. Thus the recurrence rate of

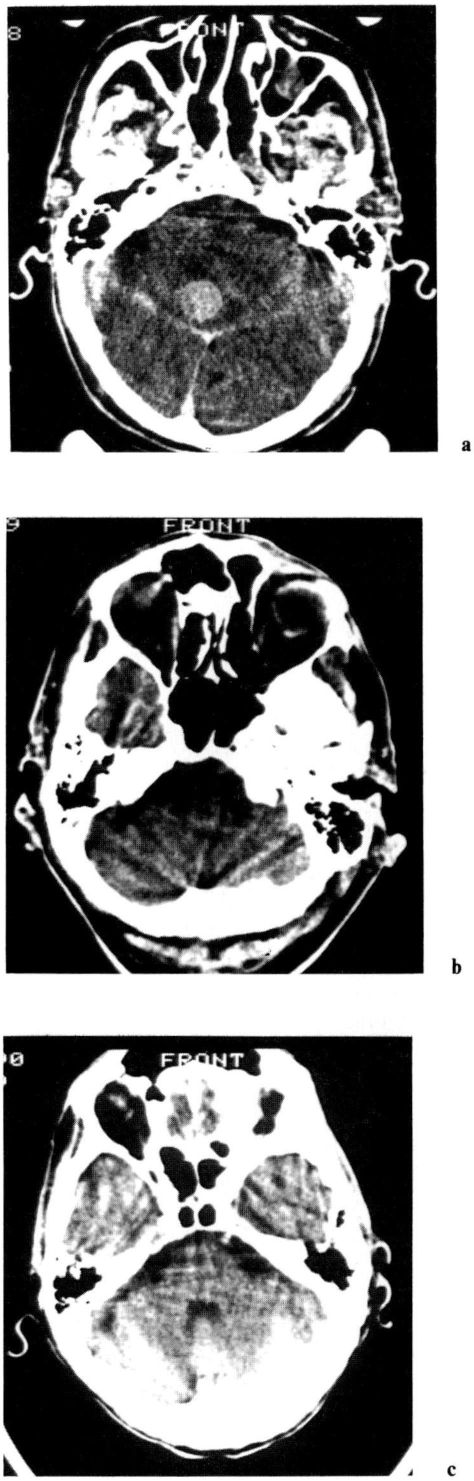

Fig. 2. Transaxial contrast-enhanced CT scans obtained prior to (a), 3 months (b), and 1 year (c) after Gamma Knife surgery in case #2

about 20% is fairly high. Better results have, however, been achieved using computer-assisted stereotactic resection of metastatic tumours[2]. Surgery is recommended only in patients with single metastasis located in a location accessible without incurring major neurological deficits to the patient. Only about 50% of metastasis are single and of those only half are accessibly located[9]. Furthermore, a limited life expectancy or poor general condition of the patient may further restrict the utility of the best available treatment i.e. surgery in combination with WBRT. Consequently, only a small minority of patients with cerebral metastases can benefit from optimal therapy. A drawback of WBRT is also the considerable amount of time consumed for the patient and the discomforts frequently caused by the therapy.

Admittedly, the observation times of patients treated by Gamma Knife surgery for metastases are short but it is nevertheless justified to conclude that this new treatment modality appears to circumvent many of the disadvantages of the conventional therapy and to increase the number of patients to which effective therapy with minimal risk can be offered.

References

1. Cairncross JG, Posner JB (1983) The management of brain metastases. In: Walker MD (ed) Oncology of the nervous system. Martinus Nijhoff, Boston, pp 341–377
2. Kelly PJ, Kall BA, Goerss SJ (1988) Results of computed tomography-based computer-assisted stereotactic resection of metastatic intracranial tumours. Neurosurgery 22: 7–17
3. Lindquist C (1989) Gamma Knife surgery for recurrent solitary metastasis of a cerebral hypernephroma: Case report. Neurosurgery 25: 802–804
4. Lindqvist C, Steiner L (1988) Radiosurgery in the treatment of arteriovenous malformations. In: Lunsford LD (ed) Modern stereotactic neurosurgery. Martinus Nijhoff, Boston, pp 491–505
5. Patchell RA, Cirrincione C, Thaler HT, *et al* (1986) Single brain metastases: Surgery plus radiation or radiation alone. Neurology 36: 447–453
6. Patchell RA, Tibbs PA, Walsh JW, Dempsey RJ, Maruyama Y, Kryscio RJ, Markesbery, WR, MacDonald JS and Young B (1990) A randomized trail of surgery in the treatment of single metastases to the brain. N Engl J Med 322: 494–500
7. Steiner L (1986) Radiosurgery in cerebral arteriovenous malformations. In: Flamm E, Fein J (eds) Textbook of cerebrovascular surgery. Springer, New York, pp 1161–1215
8. Sturm V, Kober B, Höver K-H, Schlegel W, Boesecke R, Pastyr O, Hartmann GH, Schabbert S, zum Winkel K, Kunze S, Lorenz WJ (1987) Stereotactic percutaneous single dose irradiation of brain metastases with a linear accelerator. Int J Radiat Oncol Biol Phys 13: 279–282
9. Young B, Patchell RA (1990) Surgery for a single brain metastasis. In: Wilkins RH, Rengachary SS (eds) Neurosurgery. McGraw Hill, New York, pp 473–476

Correspondence: L. Kihlström Department of Neurosurgery, Karolinska Hospital, Box 60500, S-10401 Stockholm, Sweden.

Acta Neurochirurgica, Suppl. 52, 90–92 (1991)

Solitary Brain Metastasis: Radiosurgery in Lieu of Microsurgery in 32 Patients

R.J. Coffey[1], **J.C. Flickinger**[3], **L.D. Lunsford**[2,3], and **D.J. Bissonette**[2]

[1] Department of Neurologic Surgery, Mayo Clinic/Mayo Medical School, and the [2] Department of Neurological Surgery, and [3] Radiation Oncology, The University of Pittsburgh

Summary

Thirty-two consecutive patients with 34 small brain metastases underwent boost stereotactic radiosurgery using the first North American Gamma Unit between May 1988 and July 1990. The majority of tumors (n = 24; 71%) were considered resistant to conventional, fractionated irradiation (malignant melanoma, n = 13; non-small cell lung carcinoma, n = 7; renal cell carcinoma, n = 4). During the follow-up period (median = 10 months; range = 1.5–15 months) no patient suffered a complication of radiosurgical treatment, and no patient died from a radiosurgically-treated metastasis. Shrinkage or growth-arrest was documented in 20 of 23 patients (87%) available for follow-up. Median survival after treatment was 10 months.

Keywords: Brain metastasis; brain tumor; gamma knife; radiosurgery.

Introduction

Stereotactic radiosurgery is an effective treatment alternative for selected patients with small intracranial vascular malformations or circumscribed, histologically benign extra-axial neoplasms[1,2,4,5,8,9,11]. Recent studies have indicated that stereotactic radiosurgery, using a variety of instruments, stops the growth of newly-diagnosed or recurrent brain metastases[3,6,7,12]. The present report describes our experience using the first North American 201-source cobalt-60 gamma knife to treat small, solitary brain metastases at the time of initial diagnosis ("boost radiosurgery") or at the time of recurrence after surgical resection and/or conventional fractionated irradiation.

Methods and Material

Between May 1988 to July 1990, we treated 32 consecutive patients with 34 small brain metastases using the Leksell Gamma Unit at the University of Pittsburgh. The primary tumors included malignant melanoma (n = 13), non-small cell lung carcinoma (NSCLC; n = 7), renal cell carcinoma (n = 4), colorectal carcinoma (n = 1), oropharyngeal carcinoma (n = 1), choriocarcinoma (n = 1), lymphoma (n = 1), and metastatic adenocarcinoma of unknown origin (n = 3). All tumors were solitary and ⩽ 3.0 cm in largest diameter at the time of initial presentation. A single patient with metastatic renal-cell carcinoma was treated for two new, bilateral parietal lobe tumors 10 months after successful obliteration of his original, solitary metastasis. The clinical features of the patients and the locations of the brain metastases are summarized in Tables 1 and 2.

Twenty-eight patients (30 tumors) received a planned combination of 30–40 Gy fractionated whole brain radiation therapy (WBRT) plus a single-fraction radiosurgical "boost" of 16–20 Gy to the tumor margin. Thirty two tumors (97%) were enclosed within the 50–90% isodose shells of the radiosurgical treatment plan. Three patients with NSCLC and one patient with choriocarcinoma were treated for recurrent (n = 2), persistent (n = 1), or new solitary brain metastasis (n = 1) between 6 and 20 months after conventional

Table 1. *Clinical Features of 32 Patients with Brain Metastasis Treated Using Radiosurgery*

Sex		Age (years)		Neurologic Deficit	Karnofsky Rating	
Male	Female	Mean	(Range)		Mean	(Range)
25	7	52	(24–81)	18 (56%)	80	(50–100)

Table 2. *Location of 34 Brain Metastases Treated Using Radiosurgery*

	Number	(Percent)
Lobar	22[a]	(65)
Intraventricular	1	(3)
Brainstem	8	(23)
Cerebellum	3	(9)
Total	34	(100)

[a] Left hemisphere, n = 11; right hemisphere, n = 11.

Table 3. *Results of Radiosurgery in Patients with Brain Metastasis (follow-up = 1.5–15 months)*

Tumor Size[a] (n = 23)			Neurologic Status (n = 28)			
Absent or Decreased	No Change	Increased	Improved	Stable	Worse	Dead
13	7	3[b]	6	8	2[b]	12[c]

[a] MRI or CT imaging (n = 21), or post-mortem examination (n = 2).
[b] Two patients underwent craniotomy and tumor resection 5–6 months after radiosurgery and were temporarily worse before surgery.
[c] All deaths were due to systemic disease or new, remote CNS metastasis.

external beam irradiation doses of 30–66 Gy. They received a radiosurgical dose of 12–18 Gy to the tumor margin. One patient with a metastatic renal-cell carcinoma in the third ventricle refused WBRT and was treated with radiosurgery only. High-resolution stereotactic computed tomographic (CT) and magnetic resonance imaging (MRI) were employed for target coordinate determination and treatment planning. The irradiation fields were tailored to the shape of the tumor margins using one isocenter (n = 30), two isocenters (n = 3), or three isocenters (n = 1) with the 18 mm (n = 16), 14 mm (n = 18) or 8 mm (n = 5) collimators.

Results

Patients have been followed clinically for between 1.5 and 15 months. No patient has died from growth of a radiosurgically-treated metastasis. Follow-up imaging studies (n = 21) or post-mortem examination (n = 2) documented disappearance or shrinkage of the lesion in 13 patients, and tumor necrosis or growth-arrest in 7 patients (Table 3).

Neither imaging nor post-mortem studies were available in 3 patients who died from non-neurologic causes between 3 to 7 weeks after radiosurgery. Follow-up imaging studies were still pending in 6 recently-treated patients. Complete disappearance or dramatic shrinkage of 2 renal-cell metastases occurred between 3 and 20 months after treatment. Melanomas either disappeared (n = 2), decreased in size (n = 5), or had not grown (n = 6) during follow-up as long as 15 months. Metastatic adenocarcinomas of unknown origin also dramatically decreased in size as early as 6 weeks after radiosurgery. Metastases from NSCLC were less likely to shrink (2 of 7 tumors). Two patients with NSCLC required craniotomy and tumor resection 5 and 6 months, respectively, after radiosurgery. Surgical specimens showed a combination of necrotic and viable neoplastic cells, but no pathologic changes outside the radiosurgical treatment volume.

Twelve patients died between 1 week and 10 months after radiosurgery from progression of systemic disease (n = 10) or new central nervous system metastases (n = 2). Eighteen patients were alive and relatively independent at home (Karnofsky rating ≧ 60) between 1.5 and 15 months after treatment. Median survival after radiosurgery has been 10 months to date; the one-year actuarial survival was 33.3 percent. Although the number of patients with each type of primary tumor was small, the survival data suggested that patients with advanced NSCLC were at increased risk of early death or late treatment failure.

Discussion

In our experience, stereotactic radiosurgery using the gamma knife has controlled the growth of small brain metastases regardless of tumor histology, location, prior treatment, or "resistance" to conventional irradiation. Post mortem examination showed extensive necrosis within the treatment volume 2.5 weeks after radiosurgery of a metastasis from colorectal adenocarcinoma, but no tumor necrosis one week after treatment of a renal cell carcinoma [13]. Study of a larger number of cases will be required to determine the relative significance of irradiation dosage, time interval after treatment, and tumor radiation sensitivity to account for these findings.

While the early results of radiosurgery have been encouraging, further study is needed before routine use of the technique to treat multiple lesions can be recommended. We believe that the expanded use of stereotactic techniques, especially radiosurgery, may potentially eliminate the risk of operative mortality and neurologic morbidity in patients with small, solitary brain metastases [10].

References

1. Altschuler EM, Lunsford LD, Coffey RJ, *et al* (1989) Gamma knife radiosurgery for intracranial arteriovenous malformations in childhood and adolescence. Pediatr Neurosci 15: 53–61

2. Backlund EO, Johansson L, Sarby B (1972) Studies on craniopharyngiomas. Acta Chir Scand 138: 749–759
3. Engenhart R, Kimmig B, Sturm V (1989) Stereotactically guided convergent beam irradiation of solitary brain metastases and cerebral arteriovenous malformations. In: Dyck P, Bouzaglou A (eds) Brachytherapy of brain tumors and related stereotactic Treatment Philadelphia. Hanley and Belfus, Inc., pp 119–132
4. Leksell D (1987) Stereotactic radiosurgery. Neurol Res 9: 60–68
5. Leksell L (1983) Stereotactic radiosurgery. J Neurol Neurosurg Psychiatry 46: 797–803
6. Lindquist G (1989) Gamma knife surgery for recurrent solitary metastasis of a cerebral hypernephroma: case report. Neurosurgery 25: 802–804
7. Loeffler JS, Kooy AM, Wen PY, *et al* (1990) The treatment of recurrent brain metastases with stereotactic radiosurgery. J Clin Oncol 8: 576–582
8. Lunsford LD, Flickinger J, Coffey RJ (1990) Stereotactic gamma knife radiosurgery. Initial North American experience in 207 patients. Arch Neurol 47: 169–175
9. Noren G, Arndt J, Hindmarsh T (1983) Stereotactic radiosurgery in cases of acoustic neurinoma; Further experiences. Neurosurgery 13: 12–22
10. Patchell RA, Tibbs PA, Walsh JW, *et al* (1990) A randomized trial of surgery in the treatment of single metastases to the brain. N Engl J Med 322: 494–500
11. Steiner L (1985) Treatment of arteriovenous malformations by radiosurgery. In: Wilson CB, Stein BM (eds) Cerebrovascular surgery, Vol 4. Springer, New York, pp 1161–1251
12. Sturm V, Kober B, Hover KH, *et al* (1987) Stereotactic percutaneous single dose irradiation of brain metastases with a linear accelerator. Int J Radiat Oncol Biol Phys 13: 279–282
13. Thompson BG, Coffey RJ, Flickinger JC, *et al* (1990) Stereotactic radiosurgery of small intracranial tumors: Neuropathological correlation in three patients. Surg Neurol 33: 96–104

Correspondence: R.J. Coffey, Department of Neurologic Surgery, Mayo Clinic, 200 First Street S. W., Rochester, MN 55905, USA.

Acta Neurochirurgica, Suppl. 52, 93–95 (1991)

Radiosurgical Treatment of low flow Carotid-Cavernous Fistulae

J.L. Barcia-Salorio[1,2], **F. Soler**[3], **G. Hernandez**[4], and **J.A. Barcia**[1,2]

[1] Servicio de Neurocirugia, Hospital Clinico Universitario, Valencia,
[2] Departamento de Cirurgia, Universidad de Valencia, Spain
[3] Servicio de Radiologia, Hospital Clinico Universitario, Valencia,
[4] Servicio de Terapeutica Fisica, Hospital Clinico Universitario, Valencia, Spain

Summary

The good results obtained by stereotactic radiosurgery in arteriovenous malformations has led the authors to expect similar results in low flow carotid-cavernous fistulae. In this paper, 20 cases who underwent radiosurgery with a conventional gamma source are presented. The total dose delivered was 36 to 40 Gy. 90% of the patients were cured after radiosurgery after a mean time of 7 months. Those presenting a mild improvement after a mean time of 2 months and those with a marked improvement after 4 months.

Keywords: Carotid-cavernous fistulae; arteriovenous malformation; stereotactic radiosurgery.

Introduction

The ideal treatment of carotid-cavernous fistulae (CCF) would consist of its occlusion while preserving the patency of the carotid artery.

CCF can be classified either as high flow fistulae, corresponding mainly to Parkinsons's type I, which are due to the rupture of the intracavernous carotid wall or a low flow fistulae, which include most of the Parkinson's type II fistulae. In the latter form a branch of the intracavernous carotid artery is the source of fistulous flow[5]. There is an other type in which the communication depends on a preexisting arterio-venous malformation (AVM) between the cavernous sinus and a dural branch of the internal or external carotid arteries, described by Taptas[7]. The good results of radiosurgery on cerebral AVMs[3,6] led us to believe in the success of this technique in the closure of low flow CCFs[1].

Clinical Material and Methods

Since 1977, 20 CCF have been irradiated. These include 13 spontaneous, low flow CCF (Parkinson's type I), 1 spontaneous high flow CCF (Parkinson's type I) secondary to an Ehlers-Danlos' syndrome, 3 dural AVMs, 2 post-traumatic high flow fistulae (Parkinson's type I), and iatrogenic CCF secondary to percutaneous thermocoagulation of the Gasserian ganglion, which was shown angiographically to be of low flow. In all high flow fistulae, a previous internal carotid trapping had reduced the flow in the CCF, but had not achieved its closure or the reversal of symptoms.

The stereotactic radiosurgical technique consisted of attachment of the stereoguide to a conventional Cobalt Unit, as has previously been reported 1. Irradiation was performed with a 5 mm diameter collimator and a 10 mm diameter collimator in the case of dural AVMs. A total dose of 36 to 40 Gy was delivered in all cases. A second irradiation with a dose of 40 Gy was performed in 2 cases.

Results

The results are summarized in Table 1. There was complete closure of the CCF in 90% of cases. Improvement began at a mean time of 1.6 months. It was defined as the amelioration of the main symptoms, (exophthalmos, diplopia, ptosis, visual disturbance or facial pain). Good improvement, defined as disappearance of the main symptoms, but persistence of any minor sign (conjunctival injection, tinnitus or cranial bruit) appeared after a mean time of 4 months. Clinical cure was achieved after a mean time of 7 months. In two cases, temporary reappearance of symptoms occurred after moderate improvement 2 and 12 months respectively after irradiation, but they

Table 1. *Summary of Cases and Results of Radiosurgery of CCF. Evolution Time is Expressed in Months*

Case	Age	Sex	Type	Prev. evol.	Date of operation	Dose (Gy)	Improvement begins	Frank Improv.	Curation	Recidive
1	65	F	II	10	11–77	40	0.5	1	2	
2	56	M	II	14	10–79	40	2	5	6	
3	58	F	II	6	2–80	40	2	9	12	
4	68	F	II	16	1–81	40	1	4	6	
5	71	F	II	24	8–81	40	3	6	12	
6	69	F	II	5	7–83	36	0.5	1	2	
7	64	F	II	17	12–83	36	2	4	6	
8	59	F	II	12	12–83	36	0.5	2	3	
9	46	M	I	3	1–84	36	1	6	8	2
10	36	F	II	24	4–84/5–85	36/40				
11	71	F	II	4	6–84	36	0.5	1	3	
12	81	F	AVM	15	6–84	40	2	4	6	
13	47	M	AVM	20	1–85	40	6	15	20	12
14	63	F	AVM	7	3–85/11–85	40/40				
15	57	F	II	19	11–86	40	0.5	1.5	2	
16	62	F	II	4	4–87	30	0.5	2	4	
17	59	F	II	8	6–89	30	2	4	10	
18	18	M	Iatrogenic, low flow	5	7–87	40	2	4	6	
19	19	M	I	3	2–86	40	1	3	6	
20	48	M	I	15	11–86	40	2	4	8	

regressed and disappeared in 6 and 8 months respectively. In all cured cases, a control angiogram showed total resolution.

Of the two persisting fistulae, one was a spontaneous type II fistulae, and one a dural AVM fed from an external carotid branch. In this latter case, the target had been directed to the cavernous sinus and a subsequent intraarterial embolization did not achieve closure. The patient is presently receiving stereotactic fractioned radiotherapy.

Discussion

According to classical anatomy of the cavernous sinus the carotid artery is completely surrounded by the venous blood. A CCF would be present as a result of direct rupture of the carotid wall without concomitant venous injury[2]. In contrast, Parkinson[5] reported the existence of a venous plexus surrounding the artery so that for a CCF to be produced there must be a simultaneous defect in the arterial and venous walls. Parkinson classified the CCFs in two groups; in type I CCF, a traumatic or spontaneous rupture of the carotid wall (aneurysm, collagen disease) results in a single source of blood flow feeding the fistula. This type of fistulae, can be easily closed by intraarterial embolization[8], but this frequently implies obstruction to internal carotid flow. Most of these fistulae have a high flow and spontaneous cure occurs in less than 10 per cent of cases.

In type II fistulae, a rupture is produced in an intracavernous branch of the internal carotid artery. The extensive arterial anastomoses from dural branches produce several sources, making this type of CCF more difficult to obliterate from the internal carotid artery. A third group would be represented by reopening of pre-existing dural AVMs between the cavernous sinus and dural branches from the external or internal carotid arteries. These fistulae are also difficult to obliterate intraarterialy. Type II and AVM fistulae are both of low flow and show a certain tendency to spontaneous remission[2]. As Nukui *et al.*[4] have stated, the regression of symptoms can be expected in spontaneous (mainly low-flow) fistulae between 6 months to 6 years, and accordingly, non invasive treatment is basically recommended. Although the prognosis in this type of fistulae is benign, orbital pain, tinnitus, blepharoptosis, echmosis, increase of intraoccular pressure with visual loss, failure in occular movements or simple cosmetic considerations deserve surgical consideration. The benign prognosis of this group of fistulae calls for the least invasive treatment. Radiosurgery is a bloodless, non invasive method, with minimal risks associated, so it may be the treatment of choice for low flow fistulae.

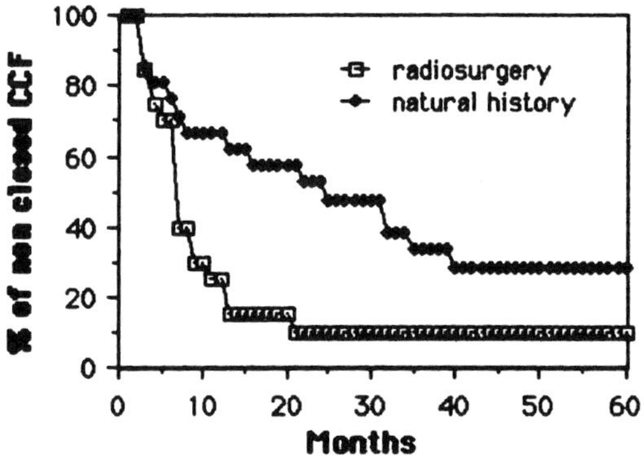

Fig. 1. Comparison between the evolution of irradiated CCF and the natural history of untreated CCF, expressed as the percentage of fistulae still unclosed at a certain time

One objection that may be made to the results reported is that obliteration after radiosurgery could reflect spontaneous closure, independent from treatment. We have studied the evolution of the cases reported by Nukui *et al.*[4] and it can be shown that the expected probability of spontaneous closure at any time is practically constant (20 months, with a standard error of 0.22). This implies that spontaneous closure of a low flow CCF is a completely random phenomenon. If this is true, the expected probability of closure for a CCF at the time of irradiation would correspond to 20 months, while our results give an expected probability of closure of 6.7 months. Figure 1 represents the percentage of non-closed CCF as a function of time, compared to what would be expected from the natural history of untreated spontaneous CCF.

Another important feature of radiosurgery is that it can be combined with a more invasive treatment (e.g., previous trapping) in case of the treatment of high flow CCF.

References

1. Barcia Salorio JL, Hernandez G, Broseta J (1982) Radiosurgical treatment of carotid-cavernousd fistulae. Appl Neurophysiol 45: 520–522
2. Day Al, Rhoton, AL (1990) Aneurysms and arteriovenous fistualae of the intracavernous carotid artery and its branches. In: Youmans JR (ed) Neurological surgery. Saunders Co., Philadelpia WB pp 1807–1863
3. Kjellberg RN, Hanumura T, Davis KR, Lyons SR, Adams AD (1983) Bragg peak proton-beam therapy for arteriovenous malformations of the brain. Engl J Med 309: 269–274
4. Nukui H, Shibasaki T, Kaneko M, Sasaki H, Mitsuka S (1984) Long-Term observations with spontaneous carotid-cavernous fistulas. Surg Neurol 21: 543–552
5. Parkinson D (1965) A surgical approach to the cavernous portion of the carotid artery. Anatomical studies and case report J Neurosurg 23: 474–483
6. Steiner L, Lindquist CH (1987) Radiosurgery in cerebral arteriovenous malformations. In: Tasker R (ed) Stereotactic surgery, Vol 2, Hanley & Belfus, Philadelpia, p 335
7. Taptas JN (1963) Arteriovenous aneurysm in pulsating exophtalmos: a new conception of the mechanism. Excerpta Medica International Congress Series 60. Amsterdam Excerpta Medica, pp 98–99
8. Vinuela F, Fox AJ, DeBrun GM, Peerless SJ, Drake CG (1984) Spontaneous carotid-cavernous fistulas: Clinical radiological and therapeutic considerations. J Neurosurg 60: 976–984

Correspondence: J.L. Barcia-Salorio, Servicio de Neurochrirurgia, Hospital Clinico Universitario, Av. Blasco Ibanez 17, E-46010 Valencia, Spain.

Movement Disorder

Acta Neurochirurgica, Suppl. 52, 99–102 (1991)

Assessing Outcome of Stereotactic and Functional Neurosurgery for Clinical Audit

C.H.A. Meyer and **E.R. Hitchcock**

Department of Neurosurgery, University of Birmingham, UK

Summary

Audit of all types of stereotactic and functional neurosurgery can be based on outcome described as a profile of changes in four parameters – symptoms/signs, overall disability, complications, and the success of surgery in eliminating neuropathology.

Keywords: Audit; disability; complications; prognosis; movement disorders; trigeminal neuralgia; extracranial pain brain gliomas.

Introduction

Doctors concerned with stereotactic and functional neurosurgery have an obligation to provide quality assurance of their clinical practice. This, an issue of great moment to authorities who fund health-care, is achieved best by audit of the outcome of management[1]. For this purpose outcome may be described as a profile of changes in four parameters:

1) The symptoms/signs for which the patient is treated,
2) The underlying neuropathological process,
3) Overall disability, and
4) Adverse clinical changes.

This assessment is demonstrated with reference to consecutive patients treated by stereotactic and functional neurosurgery and assessed at the end of inpatient care.

Methods

For these patients, all of whom had operative treatment, the outcome was assessed as follows:

(S): The change in clinical features confined to the signs and symptoms for which operation was performed (e.g. for parkinsonism, the change in tremor contralateral to thalamotomy but disregarding other symptoms/signs or coexisting disease). Rating: improvement (complete +2, incomplete +1); no change (0); deterioration (any −1, marked −2); death (−9);

(P): An operation's achievement for the disease process being treated. Rating: process eliminated (completely +3, incompletely +2); other result (+1); no operation (0);

(A): Presence at discharge of clinical complications (however slight);

(D): Disability – as performance rated on Karnofsky scale[2], an 11 point scale ranging from 0 (death) to 100 (normal, no symptoms/signs of disease). This is based on activities of daily living and takes account of presenting and coexisting conditions, any postoperative discomfort, and iatrogenic complications.

Outcome was assessed at the end of inpatient episodes for the treatment of involuntary movement (N 129), trigeminal neuralgia (133), intractable extracranial pain (79), and brain glioma (62). Operations are listed in legends to Figs. 1–3.

Results

The outcome of surgery is shown for individual patients – Fig. 1 (thalamotomy for involuntary movement) and Fig. 2 (trigeminal neuralgia) – and is summarized in Fig. 3 for groups of patients treated for involuntary movement, trigeminal neuralgia, extracranial pain, and brain gliomas.

The technical result of surgery was coded as P+1 for all patients treated by rhizotomy and functional CNS ablations, P+3 for two patients with trigeminal neuralgia treated by microvascular decompression and, for glioma patients treated by stereotactic means (Fig. 3), P+1 for surgery limited to biopsy and P+2 for substantial though incomplete reduction of mass lesions (by cyst aspiration or open tumour excision).

Clinical complications evident at the end of inpatient management (A) were usually instances of localized analgesia (following radiofrequency trigeminal rhizotomy) or features signifying disorder in the vicinity of CNS ablations (for functional procedures) or at the site of gliomas subjected to surgery. Often

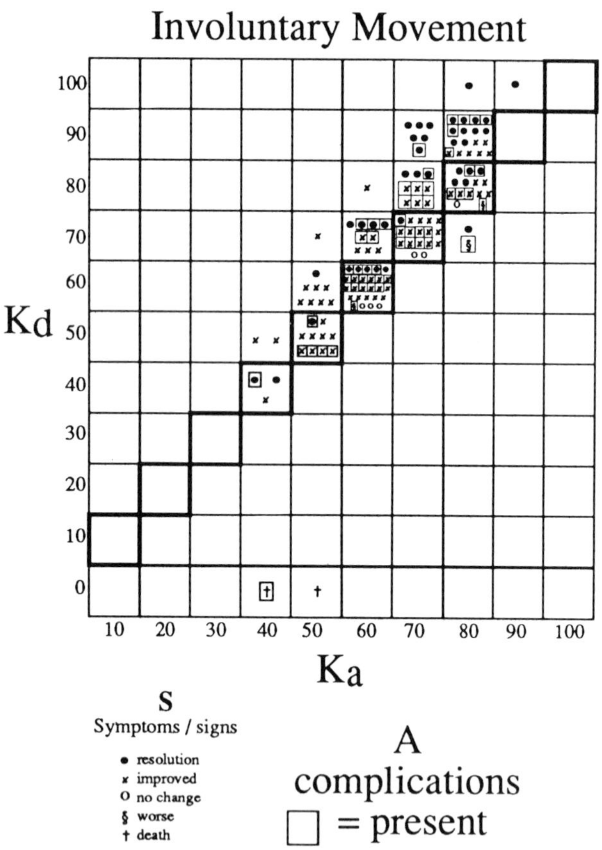

Fig. 1. Thalamotomy for Involuntary Movement. Outcome at end of 129 inpatient episodes – thalamotomy for parkinsonian tremor (33), tremor of other causes (42), chorea, athetosis, dystonia, hemiballism (18), torticollis or torsion dystonia (36) – plotted according to disability (Karnofsky score) at beginning (K_a) and end (K_d) of inpatient episode

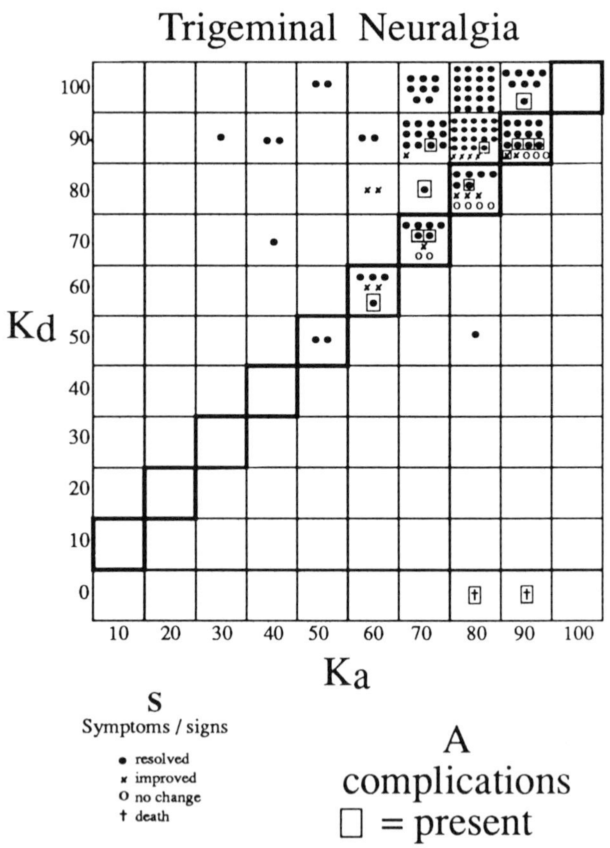

Fig. 2. Operative Treatment for Trigeminal Neuralgia. Outcome at end of 133 inpatient episodes involving treatment by radiofrequency trigeminal rhizotomy (126), injection of hypertonic saline into Meckel's cave (1), balloon compression of trigeminal ganglion (1), peripheral nerve procedures (3), and microvascular decompression (2). Individual subjects plotted according to disability (Karnofsky score) at beginning (K_a) and end (K_d) of inpatient episode

these adverse developments, especially if complicating functional operations, were mild, temporary, and would not have been evident if outcome had been assessed later at follow-up.

Adverse clinical changes (A) may coincide with improvements (S+2, +1) in symptoms/signs for which a patient is admitted and with improvement in disability rating on the Karnofsky scale (K-score) Figs. 1, 2. Note, too that changes in the symptoms/signs being treated (S+2, +1, −1) and iatrogenic complications (A) may be insufficient to cause changes in disability rating (K-score).

A general pattern of outcome was common to all three patient groups – involuntary movement, trigeminal neuralgia, extracranial pain – treated by functional neurosurgery Figs. 1–3). Usually there was improvement (S+2, +1) in the symptoms/signs for which operation was performed and improvement or no change in the disability rating (K-score): deterioration in S or in the K-score was rare. Adverse changes (A) were not uncommon but usually were mild and clinically acceptable.

For brain gliomas improvement in clinical features (S) and in disability (K-score) and the occurrence of complications were all more common after procedures coded P+2 (reduction of mass lesion) than after those coded P+1 (stereotactic biopsy only) – Fig. 3.

Discussion

This method of recording outcome is valuable for the audit of stereotactic and functional neurosurgery. It allows audit to deal with the quality of neurosurgical care rather than merely with its quantity (such as the numbers of patients treated for specified diagnoses). The four outcome parameters, S, P, A, D are easy to determine and are applicable to all neurosurgical conditions.

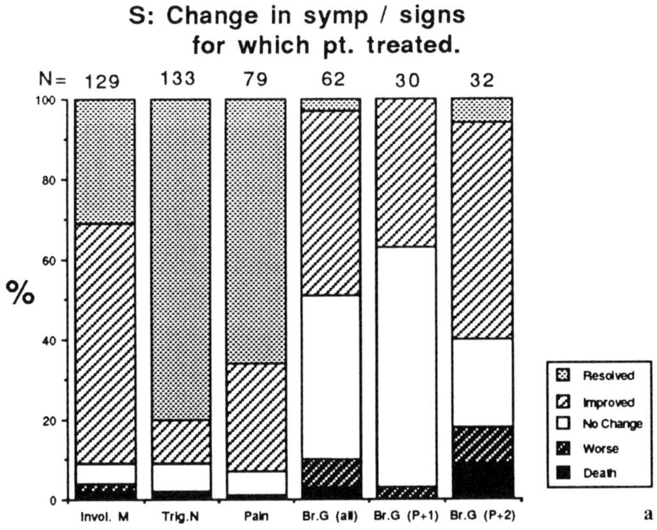

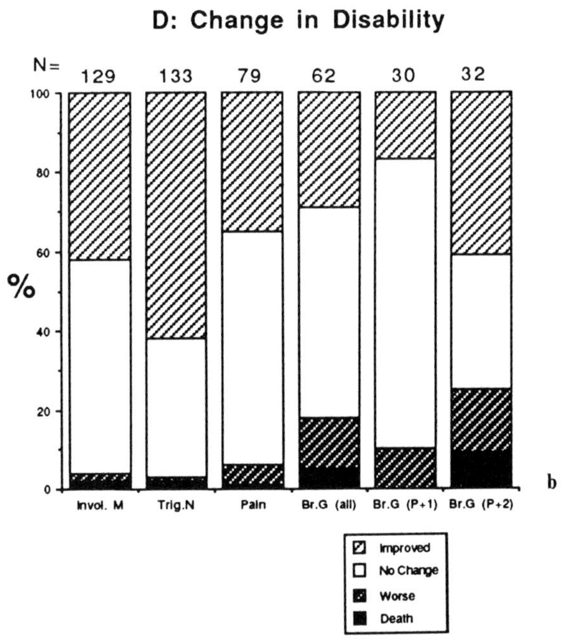

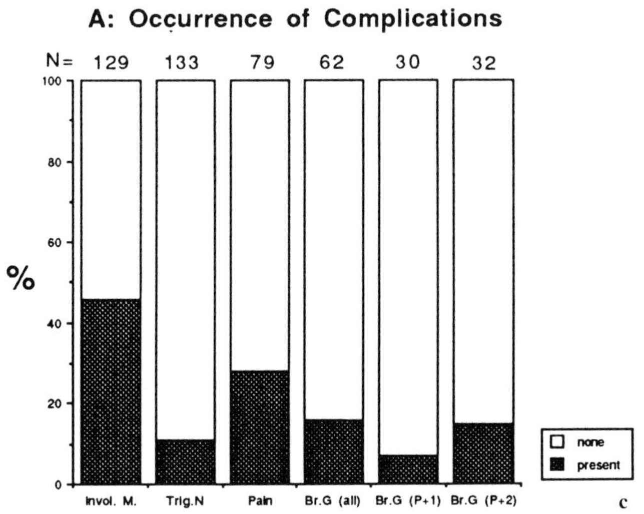

Fig. 3. Outcome of Operative Treatment assessed at end of inpatient episodes (Number: N) for (a) thalamotomy for involuntary movement (legend Fig. 1); (b) trigeminal neuralgia (legend Fig. 2); (c) intractable extracranial pain, treated stereotactically by thalamotomy N14, pontine tractomy 17, cervical commissurotomy 8, and ventrolateral cordotomy 5, and non-stereotactically by DREZ lesions 13, or spinal dorsal rhizotomy 22; and (d) brain gliomas treated stereotactically by burrhole biopsy only (P +1, N 30), burrhole biopsy and aspiration cystic glioma (P +2, N 11), or craniotomy and excision (P +2, N 21). For definition of S, D, A, P – see "Methods"

The assessment, S, allows audit to address the expectation that treatment should improve the clinical features that bring patients into neurosurgical care.

Outcome for overall disability D, is of particular concern to patients, health planners and politicians since it relates directly to a patient's capacity for domestic, recreational and vocational activities and to his need for domestic and community support services and for continued health care. For routine audit it is especially useful to rate overall disability by the Karnofsky scale[2]. This scale has gained wide acceptance over 40 years, is used readily by clinicians, and has good correlation with a subject's emotional well-being, social function and physical function[3]. Most importantly, it gives a good spread of interval points to cover the wide range of disabilities among patients managed in a general neurosurgical practice. The K-score on admittance (K_a) allows patients to be grouped according to the severity of disability at the beginning of inpatient management.

Recording clinical complications (A) allows them to be identified at audit – one aim of which is to reduce the future incidence and severity of adverse developments.

The parameter, P, denoting the technical accomplishment of surgery in eliminating or suppressing the disease process responsible for the symptoms/signs being treated, is relevant to a patient's prognosis. Moreover as a record of the type of treatment given (e.g. burrhole biopsy or operative resection of a tumour) P can help the appraisal of the other outcome parameters, S, A, and D.

All four outcome parameters should be used routinely for all patients when outcome is recorded for neurosurgical audit. Failure to record any one of these parameters would mean the loss to subsequent audit of important data concerning the quality of care for individual patients.

Clearly the outcome is influenced by the nature of the condition, (e.g. compare trigeminal neuralgia and brain glioma, Fig. 3), the severity of disability at the beginning of treatment (rated, for example, by K_a), and the nature of that treatment. By pooling results from neurosurgeons on a national or international basis-or by consensus among specialist groups – it should be possible to define standards of outcome that correspond to acceptable management for groups of patients with specified conditions. Regular review, conducted annually for example, could then compare a department's results with agreed standards of good practice. Regular review can also identify sentinel events such as patient death or a deterioration that is so unexpected that an individual instance calls for specific scrutiny. An example of this for functional neurosurgery is any deterioration in S or D (K-score). Audit using this outcome assessment sets standards, identifies unacceptable results, determines their cause, and can institute necessary changes to assure the future quality of neurosurgical practice.

While the foregoing describes outcome assessment at the end of an inpatient episode the same parameters can be used for assessment at follow-up. It is also possible to expand the content of the outcome assessment to accommodate the needs of research and specific requirements of individual neurosurgeons. However, on their own the outcome parameters described here provide data that are sufficient for audit to fulfil its purpose, viz to ensure that neurosurgical practice is kept up to a satisfactory standard. Experience over 10 years at Birmingham with the outcome ratings, S,P,A and D (i.e. change in K-score) has shown that they are quick and easy to record and that they lend themselves readily to electronic storage, retrieval, and analysis for clinical audit. This method of assessment is as applicable to stereotactic and functional neurosurgery as it is to other aspects of general neurosurgical practice.

References

1. Pollock A, Evans M (1989) Surgical audit. Butterworths, London
2. Karnofsky DA, Abelmann WH, Craver LF, Burchenal JH (1948) The use of nitrogen mustards in the palliative treatment of carcinoma. Cancer 1: 634–656
3. Spitzer WH (1987) State of science 1986: Quality of life and functional status as target variables for research. J Chron Dis 40: 456–471

Correspondence: C.H.A. Meyer, Department of Neurosurgery, University of Birmingham, Midland Centre for Neurosurgery and Neurology, Holly Lane, Smethwick, Warley, West Midlands, B69 7JX, U.K.

Acta Neurochirurgica, Suppl. 52, 103–106 (1991)

Stereotactic Vim-Vo-Thalamotomy for Choreatic Movement Disorder

Y. Kawashima, A. Takahashi M. Hirato, and **C. Ohye**

Department of Neurosurgery, Gunma University, Gunma, Japan

Summary

Two cases with hemichorea and dopa induced dyskinesia (DID) were successfully treated with Vim-Vo thalamotomy. The findings of MRI and PET of these cases were variable because of the difference of their underlying disease processes. In the patients with hemichorea, high electrical activities with irregular bursts of discharge were recorded in Vo and Vim. These may be related to dysfunction of Vo underlying choreatic movement. Regardless of the causes, their choreatic movement was abolished by Vim-Vo thalamotomy affecting mainly Vo after physiological identification of Vim.

Keywords: Hemichorea; dopa induced dyskinesia; stereotactic surgery; thalamus.

Introduction

The neurophysiological mechanism of choreatic or ballistic movements is not fully understood. The pallidothalamic pathway is one of the final outputs from basal ganglia neuronal network and dysfunction of the basal ganglia is thought to play an important role in producing these movement disorders. Therefore, this system has been selected as a target for stereotactic treatment of hyperkinetic movement disorders. For example, Spiegel reported the effect of pallidotomy for treatment of choreatic movement (4). Kandel recommended combined stereotactic destruction of VL and subthalamic area (zona incerta, fields H1 and H2 of Forel) for treatment of hemihyperkinesias (1). Dopamine induced dyskinesia (DID) has both choreatic or ballistic elements. Narabayashi claimed that levodopa induced dyskinesia is a reverse phenomenon of Parkinsonian rigidity and may reflect dysfunction of the pallidothalamic pathway. He showed that DID was almost completely abolished by lesions in the Vo complex (2).

In this paper, we report two cases with hemichorea and DID who were successfully treated by stereotactic Vim-Vo thalamotomy. Findings of MRI, PET and intraoperative depth semi-microelectrode recording are also shown.

The first patient with hemichorea was a 44-year-old woman. She had an episode of asphyxia due to aspiration of food 7 months before admission. Involuntary choreatic movements of the right side started one month after this accident. She displayed intermittent choreatic movements involving the right side with pronation-supination of the arm, elevation of the shoulder and adduction of the thigh. The involuntary movements increased under emotional stress and were suppressed during voluntary movement of the affected limbs. Magnetic resonance imaging (MRI) revealed hyperdense lesions (T2-weighted) bilaterally in the palladium (Fig. 1A). Positron emission tomography (PET) showed an increase of local cerebral glucose metabolism (LCMRGlc) in the left lenticular nucleus (Fig. 1B). As drugs were ineffective, selective thalamotomy was performed using microelectrode techniques described by Ohye (3). Depth recording during the course of stereotactic thalamotomy showed irregular bursts of discharges in the left palladium and Vo, Vim nuclei (Fig. 2). The choreatic movements disappeared immediately after a coagulation of the left Vim and Vo.

The second patient with hemichorea was a 52-year-old man. He had left hemiparesis of sudden onset. MRI showed multiple infarcts including the right pallidum, head of caudate nucleus, temporal and parieto-occipital cortex (Fig. 1C). He was diagonsed as polycythemia vera on blood examination. Two months later, choreatic movements of the left upper limb became evident. He was treated by haloperidol without benefit and was admitted to our clinic one and a half after the onset.

Neurological examination revealed slight hemiparesis and hemihypesthesia on the right side. He displayed jerky choreatic movements on his right upper limb. Shaking motion of the arm and flexion and extension of the fingers were continuously observed except during sleep. The involuntary movements were exaggerated under emotional stress and suppressed during voluntary movement of the affected limb.

PET showed decrease of LCMRGlc in the right caudate nucleus (Fig. 1D).

After haematological control, stereotactic operation was performed. Irregular bursts of discharges were recorded in the right Vo, Vim nuclei by depth recording. The values of background activity were plotted in Fig. 3A (left) along two tracks parallel to the sagittal plane. The superimposed map shows the corresponding profile of the thalamus. The high electrical activity continued from

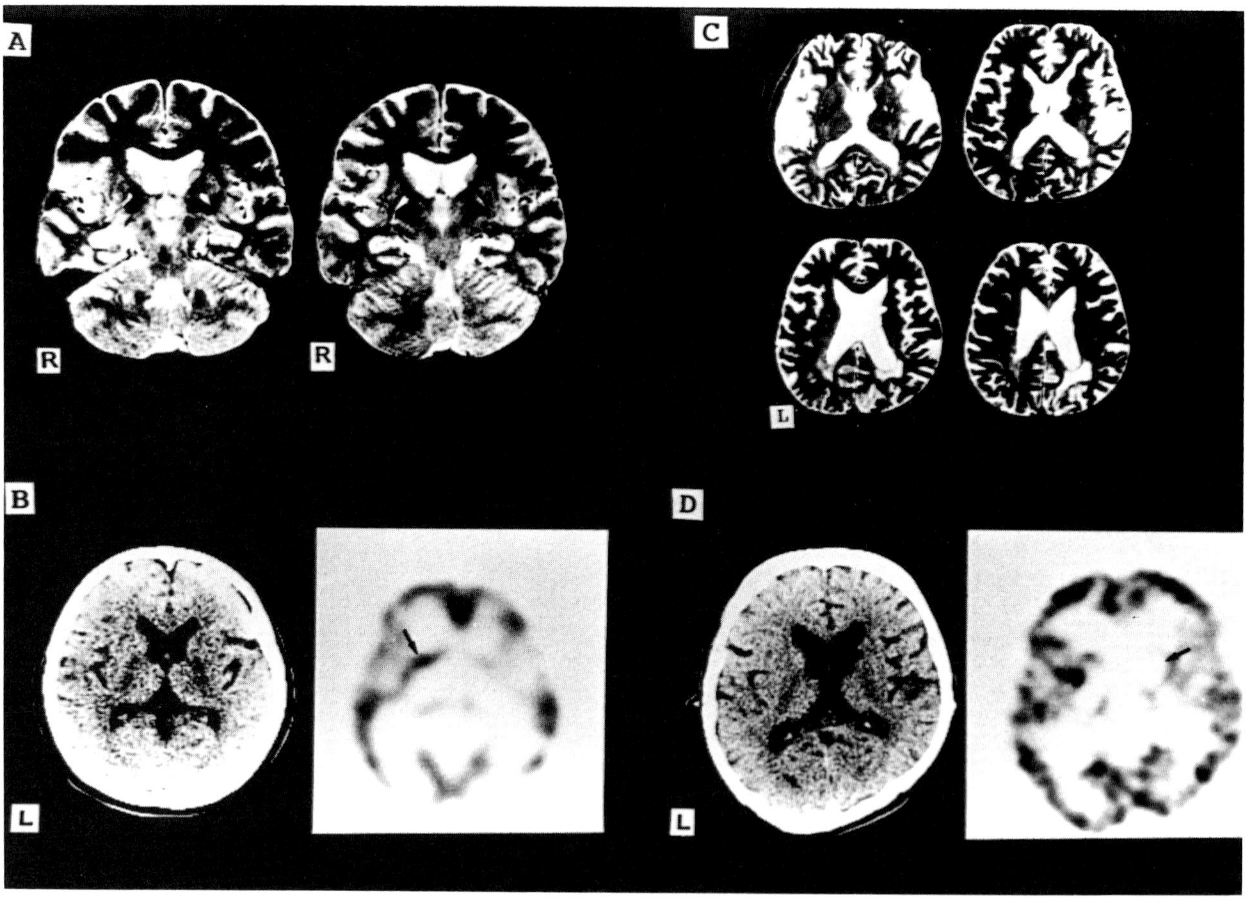

Fig. 1. MRI T2 weighted image of case 1 (A) and case 2 (C). CT and the same section of PET image (18FDG) of case 1(B) and case 2 (D)

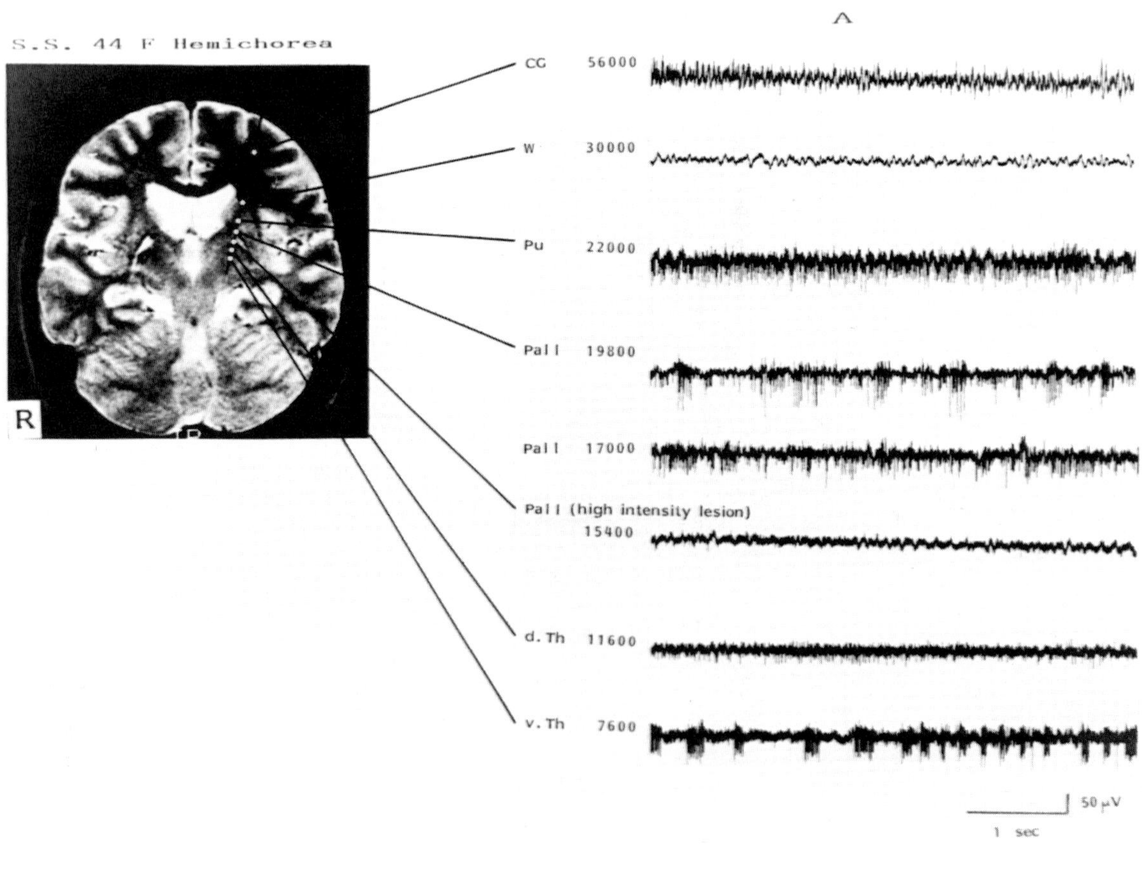

Vo to Vim. The choreatic movements completely disappeared after right Vim-Vo thalamotomy (Fig. 3A right).

The third patient was a 42-year-old man. Since five years he had been treated for Parkinson's disease with bilateral rigidity, resting tremor and hypokinesia, using l-dopa. DIDs were noted on both side since three years and gradually increased. MRI showed no abnormal findings. PET revealed increased LCMRGlu in left lenticular nucleus. Dyskinesias were absent during PET study in this patient.

The fourth case was a 48-year-old man. He had been treated as Parkinson's disease for 9 years because of rigidity, starting hesitation and frozen gait. DID, more marked on the left side, became evident one year before admission. MRI showed no abnormal findings. PET revealed increased LCMRGlu in the lenticular nuclei. In this patient,

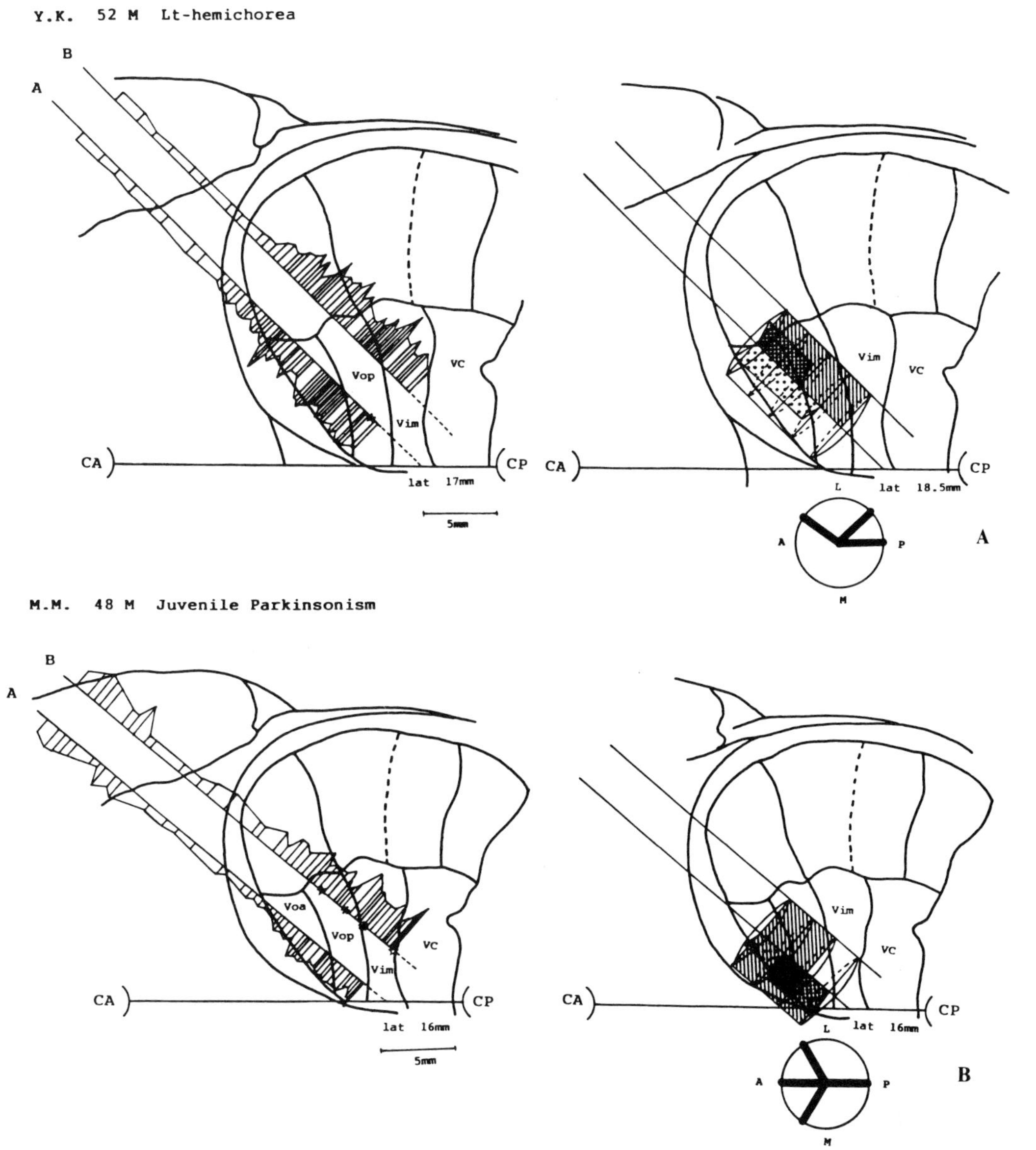

Fig. 3. The values of background activity (left) and the extent of the lesion (right) in case 2 (A) and case 4 (B). The values of electrical activity are plotted along two tracks inserted parallel to the sagittal plane. Small coagulation lesions were made in Vim and Vo. The extent of the lesion is also shown in cross-section. Superimposed maps show the corresponding profile of the human thalamus

In case 2, a kinesthetic response to movement of the jaw was recorded at the point marked by star (★).

In case 4, four kinesthetic responses were recorded: response to abduction of forearm (★), response to elbow flexion (★, ★), response to tap at the tip of the tongue (☆)

◄

Fig. 2. Depth microelectrode recording during operation of case 1. CG: cortical gray matter, W: white matter, Pu: putamen, Pall: palladium, d.Th: dorsal thalamus, v.Th: ventral thalamus, A: electrode A. The MRI image represents the same plane as the trajectory of the A-electrode. Numbers indicated on the left of electrical activity depict the distance from the tentative target point (=zero) in μm. Electrode A was directed 5 mm anterior to the posterior commissure and 15 mm lateral to the midline

high electrical background activity was recorded mainly in Vim. The DID as well as tremor and rigidity were abolished by a contralateral Vim-Vo thalamotomy. The sequential changes of neural activity along the tracks and coagulation lesions are shown in Fig. 3B.

Discussion

MRI and PET findings in these four patients with choreatic movement were variable, probably because the lesions that were either directly or indirectly responsible for the symptoms were different: ischemic cerebrovascular disease (patient 1), anoxic disease (patient 2) and Parkinson's disease (patients 3 and 4). In the patient with hemichoraea, high electrical activity with irregular bursts of discharge were recorded in Vo and Vim. This may be related to dysfunction of Vo underlying the choreatic movement. On the other hand, in the Parkinsonian patients with DID high electrical activity was recorded mainly in Vim. Regardless of the causes, the choreatic movements were abolished by Vim-Vo thalamotomy affecting mainly Vo after physiological identification of Vim nucleus.

Microelectrode technique aided by stereotactic MRI and PET is useful not only for physiological identification of the thalamic subnucleus but also to study the functional state of the subcortical structures in movement disorders.

References

1. Kandel EI (1982) Treatment of hemihyperkinesias by stereotactic operation on basal ganglia. Appl Neurophysiol 45: 225–229
2. Narabayashi H, Yokochi F, Nakajima Y (1984) Levodopa-induced dyskinesia and thalamotomy. J Neurol Neurosurg Psychiatry 47: 831–839
3. Ohye C (1988) Selective thalamotomy for movement disorders: Microrecording stimulation techniques and results. In: Lunsford LD (ed) Modern Stereotactic Neurosurgery. Boston Martinus Nijhoff, pp 315–331
4. Spiegel EA, Wycis HT (1950) Pallidothalamotomy in chorea. Arch Neurol Psychiatry 64: 295–296

Correspondence: Y. Kawashima, Department of Neurosurgery, Gunma University, 3–39–22, Showamachi, Maebashi, Gunma, Japan.

Thalamic and Dorsal Column Stimulation

Acta Neurochirurgica, Suppl. 52, 109–111 (1991)

Thalamic Stimulation for the Treatment of Tremor and Other Movement Disorders

S. Blond[1] and **J. Siegfried**[2]

[1]Department of Neurosurgery, C.H.R.U., Lille, France and [2]AMI Klinik Im Park, Zürich, Switzerland

Summary

Thalamic stimulation for the treatment of tremor and other motor movement disorders is attractive in view of the fact that it is a non-destructive procedure. With the experience of 26 cases indications can be defined. The method is an alternative for treatment of tremor only when thalamotomy carries a high risk of complications. Not only is the cost a limiting factor but also repeated operations for replacing the neuro-pacemaker and thus the risk of infection have to be taken in consideration.

Keywords: Movement disorders; tremor; thalamic stimulation; results; indication.

Introduction

Since the introduction of stereotactic brain operations for functional disorders in 1947, electrical stimulation of deep brain structures has been practised, particularly for anatomical localization. Data obtained along the 1960s showed that low frequency electrical stimulation in the ventrolateral part of the thalamus increases or even evokes tremor and/or other hyperkinetic patterns, while higher frequencies and amplitude may either augment or suppress an existing spontaneous hyperkinesia. In the 1970s deep brain stimulation was used in humans to influence movements disorders[2,3,4,9,10]. Since localized small stereotactic destruction in the VL thalamus has been recognized to suppress tremor and rigidity of Parkinson's disease and tremor of other origins in a very high percentage of cases without producing clinically detectable neurological deficits, this method remained the neurosurgical treatment of choice for tremor.

In 1980, Brice and Mc Lellan[6] reported a suppression or decrease of severe intention tremor in 3 women with multiple sclerosis by continuous stimulation of the subthalamic region. Stimulation of this region with 75–150 Hz with square wave pulses of 0.5–1.0 Oma of 200–400 ms duration was so successful that it was continued with an external radiofrequency transmitter. To reduce the total amount of stimulation delivered to the patient, the transmitter was controlled by a switching device triggered by electromyographic signals from the deltoid muscle of the appropriate arm. The transmitter was automatically switched on as soon as the deltoid muscle was activated and switched off after 5–7s.

Benabid[5] in 1987 implanted a stereotactic stimulation device in the ventrolateral part of the thalamus (nucleus Vim) to control Parkinson tremor. As an alternative to other methods, high frequency stimulation yield good results.

The experience of the authors since 1980 in dyskinesia/dystonia treated by chronic VPL stimulation and since 1987 for Parkinson tremor and others by VL stimulation is reported. The respective role of each-structure will be discussed and the advantages and disadvantages of this method emphasized.

Material and Methods

Since 1980, four cases of dyskinesia and dystonia, after post-apoplectic syndrome and since 1987, nineteen cases of Parkinsonian tremor, two cases of essential tremor and one case of complex tremor have been operated on (Table 1). A manipular electrode with control stylet was placed in VPL somatotopically to treat dyskinesia/dystonia and in the Vim for tremor. Test stimulation was followed for a few days. A screw made with pure titanium, a material highly biocompatible with bone, is used to secure the electrode in a burr hole of 2.5 mm: the screw provides also a water-tight seal of the burr hole[12]. When the tremor is satisfactory controlled, a neuropacemaker is implanted in subcutaneous pocket under lathe clavicle and connected to the electrode. The parameters of stimulation are shown in Table 2.

Table 1. *Own Series (Implanted)*

– Parkinson tremor	:	19
– Essential tremor	:	2
– Complex tremor	:	1
– Dyskinesia-dystonia	:	4

Table 2. *Method*

- Monopolar DBS Medtronic Ytrel I
- Parameters
  - VL 8 mm in front of CP
    - 0,25–1,25 (m̄: 0,75 v)
    - 210 micro sec.
    - 130 Hz
    - 60 sec. on/2 sec. off day and night
  - VL 6 mm in front of CP
    - 1.–2.75 (m̄: 1.75 v)
    - 210 micro sec.
    - 130 Hz
    - day and night: 7
    - continuous day: 6
  - VPL – 0,5–1 v (m̄: 0,68)
    - 210 micro sec.
    - 33–60 Hz (40 Hz)
    - 60 or 120 sec. on/60 sec. off

Results

Tremor

a) Parkinsonian Tremor: Of nineteen cases, twelve had an excellent result with total suppression of tremor, as long as the stimulation was on. In seven cases, the tremor was only partially controlled. In ten cases, the stimulation was continuous during the day: five of them used the stimulation also during the night since there was a massive rebound of tremor as soon as the stimulation stopped. In nine cases, of which five presented the rebound phenomenon, the neuro-pacemaker was programmed at a stimulation of 60 seconds on and two seconds off. Foot dystonia was present in two cases of this series of 19 patients. In one case, amplitude was increased to 2.5 v for total tremor control, when a dysarthia appeared, requiring a current reduction to 1.5 v.: tremor control was then less satisfactory in this case. In one case, a lateropulsion to the side of the tremor was considerable to be a side effect.

b) Essential and Complex Tremor: Total suppression of tremor was obtained only in one case of essential tremor. In the second case, the tremor was partially controlled; a rebound phenomenon required continuous stimulation. In one of the cases tremor was so poorly influenced that a high frequency coagulation was performed despite a previous thalamotomy on the other side; however, the result was excellent, without complication. One case of complex tremor has partial effect.

c) Post-Apoplectic Dyskinesia Dystonia: With VPL chronic stimulation, involuntary movements were successfully controlled in three cases and partially in one case.

Discussion

The actual place of thalamic stimulation to treat tremor and movement disorders has to be critically analyzed. The great advantage of this method is its reversibility and probably the absence of brain lesions; however, we still do not know if a continuous long-term stimulation does not produce neuronal damages. The draw-backs of the method is that it necessitates two operations, prolonged hospitalization, risk of infection and possible reject reactions. Last but not the least, cost of the device which has to be replaced after some time must be taken into account. As far as tremor is concerned, our results and those in BENABIDs larger series, show that in about 65 per cent of the patients the tremor is completely suppressed. Nevertheless, the excellent results of classical thalamotomy with permanent suppression of tremor, indicates what deep brain requiring a second thalamotomy on the dominant side in case there is speech impairment or if that complication is expected to occur together with psychoorganic disturbances.

In post-apoplectic dyskinesia/dystonia, thalamotomy is rarely indicated. In these cases, stimulations is an alternative specially when sensory disturbances are present. The only possible target must be the sensory nuclei but anatomical integrity of the region has to be controlled preoperatively with CT or MRI (Table 3).

The possible mechanism involved can only be speculated. The fact that frequencies below 100 HZ mainly increases tremor when stimulating VL and

Table 3. *Indications*

- Tremor: – Second-side after VL thal. for one side
  - Preexisting speech disturbances
  - Old patients with psycho-organic disturbances
- Dyskinesia – Dystonia:
  - In case of sensory disturbances

higher frequencies produce inhibition, may suggest that the therapeutic effect is due to an inhibition of neuronal activity. The stimulation inhibits the cells which can be destroyed by coagulation. The beneficial effects of VL thalamic stimulation could be a functional ablation of the discharging system[1].

In our series, the same satisfactory therapeutic effect has been obtained by stimulation of the Vim very close to the VPL or 2 mm in front. When the electrode tip is very near to the VPL, paresthesias are obtained: It is not clear if an effect on the VPL is necessary. The importance of VL and especially the VPL input to the motor cortex is indicated by the fact that 70% of all thalamocortical connections originates from VPL, and 95% from VLc, VIo and VPLo[11]. The physiological importance of the thalamus as an efferent relay of information from the basal ganglia and an efferent relay of revised information to the motor and premotor cortex has been emphasized[7,8]. This function of thalamic output, which modifies motor behaviour, is related to pathophysiological mechanisms in movement disorders. Examples are the inability of athetotic patients to control their movements without the help of sensory input, and the "guest antagonist" phenomenon which occurs when a patient is able to modify torticollis by lightly placing an index finger on the chin[14].

In cases of dyskinesia/dystonia with sensory deafferentation the VPL stimulation probably supply or augment the sensory activity.

References

1. Andy DJ (1983) Thalamic stimulation for control of movement disorders. Appl Neurophysiol 46: 107–111
2. Bechtereva NP, Bondartchuk AN, Smirnov VM, Meliutcheva LA (1972) Therapeutic electrostimulations of the brain deep structures. Vopr Neirokhnir 1: 7–12
3. Bechtereva NP Bondartchuk AN, Smirnov VM, Meliutcheva LA, Shandurina AN (1975) Method of electrostimulation of the deep brain structures in treatment of some chronic diseases. Confin Neurol 37: 136–140
4. Bechtereva NP, Kambarova DK, Smirnov VM, Shandurina AN (1975) Using the brain's latent abilities for therapy: chronic intracerebral electrical stimulation. In: Sweet WH, Obrador S, Martin-Rodriguez JG (eds) Neurosurgical treatment in psychiatry, pain and epilepsy. University Park Press, Baltimore London Tokyo 581–613
5. Benabid AL, Pollak P, Louveau A, Henry S, De Rougemont J (1987) Combined (thalamotomy and stimulation) stereotactic surgery of the VIM thalamic nucleus for bilateral Parkinson's disease. Proceedings of the Meeting of the American Society for Stereotactic and Functional Neurosurgery, Montreal 1987 Appl Neurophysiol 50: 344–346
6. Brice J, Mc Lellan L (1980) Suppression of intention tremor by contingent deep brain stimulation. Lancet 2: 1221–1222
7. Delong MR, Georgopoulos AP, Crutcher MD (1984) In: Function of the basal ganglia. Ciba Foundation Symposium 107. Pitman, London 64–72
8. Evarts EV, Wise SP (1984) In: Function of the basal ganglia. Ciba Foundation Symposium 107. Pitman, London 83–102
9. Mundinger F (1979) Neue stereotaktisch-funktionelle Behandlungsmethode des Torticollis spasmodicus mit Hirnstimulatoren. Med Klin 72: 1982–1986
10. Mundinger F, Neumuller H (1982) Programmed stimulation for control of chronic pain and motor disease. Appl Neurophysiol 45: 102–111
11. Porter R (1984) In: Function of the basal ganglia. Ciba Foundation Symposium 107. Pitman, London 130–107
12. Siegfried J, Comte P, Meier R (1983) Intracerebral electrode implantation system. J Neurosurg 59: 356–359
13. Siegfried J, Pamir MN (1987) Electrical stimulation in human of the sensory thalamic nuclei and effects on dyskinesias and spasticity Clinical aspects of sensory motor integration. Struppler A, Weindl A (eds) Springer, Berlin Heidelberg New York Tokyo
14. Siegfried J (1986) Effets de la stimulation du noyau sensitif du thalamus sur les dyskinésies et la spasticité. Rev Neurol 142 (4): 380–383
15. Siegfried J (1987) Stimulation of thalamic nuclei in human: Sensory and therapeutical aspects. In: Besson JM, Guilbaud G, Peschanski M (eds) Thalamus and Pain, Elsevier Science Publishers BV 271–278

Correspondence: S. Blond, Department of Neurosurgery, C.H.R.U., F-59037 Lille, France.

Acta Neurochirurgica, Suppl. 52, 112–117 (1991)

Therapeutical Neurostimulation – Indications Reconsidered

J. Siegfried

AMI Klinik Im Park, Zürich, Switzerland

Summary

A critical review of indications, limitations and results of different modalities of neurostimulation is given, based on large personal experiences since 1972 and on literature report.

Keywords: Neurostimulation; spinal root stimulation; spinal cord stimulation; thalamic stimulation; pain; movement disorders; spasticity; breathing control; bladder stimulation.

Introduction

As early as 1780, Galvani stimulated frog nerve and observed the resultant muscle twitch. Later on, electrical stimulation in the periphery, and in the central nervous system became utilized in defining brain areas and in mapping neural circuitry. The modification of functional neurological disorders through electrical neurostimulation has been early recognized, but its application as therapeutical tool became only possible with the advent of electronic stimulators that could be implanted within the body. It seemed more and more reasonable to assume that it would be safer to apply chronic neurostimulation, which could be discontinued at any time, than to perform destructive or ablative procedure which is irreversible. This new technique then went in search of indications and many nervous structures have been stimulated for many neurological disorders (Table 1). The actual place of this method has to be regularly reconsidered, and based on the literature and on our own experience of eighteen years, particularly in pain treatment, but also in the management of motor movement disorders, we will try to outline the best indications. Since the use of electrical stimulation in the treatment of chronic pain is the most common application, but still a controversial issue, we will focus on our personal experience since 1972 in this field.

I. Neurostimulation for Chronic Pain

Classification of organic pain in different categories has been the decisive factor governing pain therapy. The identification of two main forms of fundamentally different pain, nociceptive (somatogenic) and neuropathic (neurogenic, deafferentation pain), which has to be the first step before proposing a therapeutical attempt, was not recognized when the technique of dorsal cord stimulation was introduced in 1967[15]. Inaccurate indications, poor selection of patients, inappropriate levels of stimulation, inadequately

Table 1. *Overview of the Main Attempts to Correct Neurological Disorders by Chronic Stimulation of Nervous Structures*

Peripheral nerve	Foot drop	1961	Liberson
	Diaphragm pacing	1959	Glenn
	Pain	1965	Sweet
Gasserian ganglion	Pain	1980	Meyerson
Dorsal cord	Pain	1967	Shealy
	Spasticity	1973	Cook
	Circulatory disturbances	1976	Cook
Conus medullaris	Micturition	1970	Nashold
Deep brain	Psychiatric disorders	1953	Heath
	Pain	1962	Mazars
	Unconsciousness	1969	Hassler
	Involuntary movements	1973	Bechtereva
Cerebellum (cortex)	Epilepsy	1973	Cooper
	Motor movements disorders	1973	Cooper
Dentate nucleus	Spasticity	1979	Schvarcz
Cortex	Blindness	1967	Brindley

controlled studies, conflicting results and unreliable equipment led to great controversy on the value of the method. A long-term follow-up of a large series carefully analysed give us the opportunity to reevaluate the method and to propose some guide-lines for improving the rate of success.

1. Dorsal Spinal Root and Dorsal Cord Stimultation

After a couple of trials in 1972, the present study began in 1973 with the use of a pain profile, which is based on a five-grade rating score (the duration of pain, the intensity of pain with a visual analogue scale, the level of activity, the influence on mood and behavior, and the use of drugs). From May 1973 to May 1989 (follow-up of 1 to 16 years), dorsal cord and/or dorsal spinal root stimulation in the epidural space has been applied in a series of 669 consecutive patients with chronic intractable pain of different types according to the classification of Meyerson[13]: nociceptive, nociceptive-neurogenic, neurogenic, neuropathic, deafferentation pain. Each patient underwent trial stimulation for 2 to 7 days via stimulating electrodes introduced percutaneously or via a laminotomy epidurally along the dorsal cord or segmentally at the level of dorsal spinal roots corresponding to the distribution of pain. When the area of postganglionic neurogenic pain is restricted to 1 to 3 peripheral nerves, the posterior spinal roots involved will be directly stimulated. When the area of postganglionary pain involves a wider territory, the dorsal columns will be stimulated.

Of these 669 patients tested, 398 (59%) reported significant pain reduction and underwent implantation of a permanent subcutaneous receiver or, since 1983, a totally programmable neuropacemaker (ITREL Medtronic). Table 2 analyses the results according to the diagnosis. This series shows good to very good results in 65% of the cases. However, in cases of pure neurogenic pain as a result of peripheral nerve lesions 90% of the patients report very satisfactory pain relief; this indication is certainly the best one, when the nerve lesion is postganglionic (traumatic or iatrogenic) and when the pain is located in the upper extremity which permits direct stimulation of the corresponding dorsal spinal root. This particular series has been analysed separately[17]. Neuropathies (short series) and partial cord lesions have also a satisfactory outcome. Pain in cases of degenerative diseases (multiple sclerosis, amyotrophic lateral sclerosis, etc.) may be well improved at the beginning, but probably due to the progression of diseases with more and more functional disturbances in the dorsal columns, the success diminish. Postherpetic pain is a poor indication with exceptional improvements; this is probably due to the progressive loss of myelin and axons in the dorsal cord following the acute onset; however, we have recently had encouraging results when applying this technique in the first few months of the chronic pain, and not after more than 1 year. Plexus avulsion does not respond at all to dorsal cord stimulation as we reported already in 1984[10]; this is due to the cord lesion created by avulsion. Pain due to so-called "lumbosacral fibrosis" has to be evaluated with regard to the fact that such conditions generally comprise at least 2 types of pain: nociceptive and neuropathic. Radicular pain in one or both legs (nociceptive-neurogenic pain) may be

Table 2. *Long-term Results of Dorsal Cord and/or Dorsal Spinal Roots Stimulation for Chronic Intractable Brain According to Diagnosis*

(1973–1989)	Implanted	Long-term follow-up very good	good	fair	poor
Peripheral nerve lesions	127	84	32	9	2
"Lumbosacral fibrosis"	123	20	51	27	25
Degenerative diseases	56	3	18	16	19
Postherpetic	21	0	7	6	8
Phantom/Stump	19	3	10	3	3
Cord lesions (partial)	17	5	8	3	1
Plexus avulsion (until 1978)	8	0	0	0	8
Neuropathies	8	2	5	1	0
Ischemic pain	19	3	9	5	2
	398	260			138

improved in about 50% in the cases, the low back pain being almost often unchanged. Finally, ischemic pain is satisfactorily controlled in more than 60% of the cases.

This study shows clearly that neuropathic post-ganglionic pain is the best indication for dorsal cord and/or dorsal spinal roots stimulation. In this group, the failures can be explained in many cases by functional disturbance in the spinal cord. There is convincing evidence that peripheral nerve injury does induce alterations in the central nervous system[18]. Injury to the peripheral branch of a primary afferent neuron may result in transganglionic changes in the central branch including the axonal terminals within the dorsal horn. Ultrastructural evidence points to at least transganglionic degeneration, but whether this is due to cell death or to removal of a trophic influence remains controversial. There is no morphological evidence for collateral sprouting in the dorsal horn following nerve section but transsynaptic changes in second order neurons have been found. After several days the functionally denervated region of the spinal cord begins to show alterations such as expansion in the dorsal horn neuronal receptive field, so that cells that were formerly innervated exclusively by the denervated skin areas start to respond to stimuli also outside the original receptive field.[7]

2. *Sensory Thalamic Stimulation*

From March 1977 to December 1989, sensory thalamic stimulation has been applied in a series of 168 consecutive patients suffering of chronic intractable neuropathic pain. A smooth monopolar electrode with a central stylet was introduced stereotactically into the nucleus ventroposteromedialis thalamic for pain in the face, the medial part of the nucleus ventroposterolateralis for pain in the arm, and the lateral part of the nucleus ventroposterolateralis for the leg. After trial stimulation of 2 to 7 days, 119 patients (70%) reported significant pain reduction and subsequently underwent implantation of a permanent subcutaneous receiver or, since 1983, a programmable neuropacemaker (ITREL Medtronic). Long-term follow-up shows good to very good results in 68% of the cases (Table 3). According to the diagnosis, this series shows particularly good results in postherpetic facial neuralgia; failures are cases of long history of pain before the operation, implying that degeneration of the trigeminal nerve up to the nucleus ventro-posteromedialis may have occurred. This is also true for iatrogenic or traumatic anaesthesia dolorosa of the face. The relatively limited success obtained in cases of pain resulting from avulsion of the brachial plexus has been evaluated by Mazars and Choppy in their series[11]; they stated that the patients with avulsion of more than two roots and large areas of anesthesia have a very low response to thalamic stimulation. They postulated that those patients with multiple avulsions had significant dorsal horn damage with resultant thalamic lesions by ascending degeneration, and thus were less responsive to thalamic stimulation. In post-stroke pain syndrome, the success appears to depend

Table 3. *Long-term Results of Sensory Thalmic Stimulation for Neuropathic Pain According to Diagnosis*

		Long-term follow-up			
(1977–1989)	Implanted	very good	good	fair	poor
Postherpetic (Trigeminus)	25	13	5	4	3
Anesthesia dolorosa face	24	10	6	5	3
Post-stroke pain syndrome	19	5	7	3	4
Brachial plexus avulsion	15	4	4	3	4
Leg plexus avulsion	1	0	1	0	0
Phantom	13	8	2	2	1
Cancer face	6	2	3	0	1
Paraplegia	4	0	2	2	0
Hemiplegia	1	0	1	0	0
Postthoractomy	1	0	0	0	1
Neurogenic in one leg	7	2	3	1	1
Vascular pain (leg)	1	0	1	0	0
Wallenberg syndrome	1	1	0	0	0
Postcordotomy	1	1	0	0	0
	119	81		38	

Table 4. *Rate of Success of Chronic Dorsal Cord, Dorsal Spinal Roots and Sensory Thalamic Stimulation long-term follow-up for Neuropathic and Ischemic Pain*

Dorsal cord stimulation	
May 1973 – May 1989	669 patients tested 398 implants (59%)
Long-term follow-up Good – very good pain relief:	neuropathic pain: 65% ischemic pain: 63%
Sensory thalamic stimulation	
March 1977 – December 1989	168 patients tested 119 implants (70%)
Long-term follow-up Good – very good pain relief:	neuropathic pain 68%

Table 5. *The Present, best Indications and the best Targets in the Nervous System for Chronic Therapeutic Neurostimulation in Functional Neurosurgery*

I. Pain	
1. Neuropathic (neurogenic, deafferentation)	
Level of neuropathy	Structure to be preferentially stimulated
Peripheral (postganglionic) lesion of 1–3 nerves	Dorsal spinal root, epidurally (peripheral nerve, Gasserian ganglion)
Peripheral (postganglionic)	Dorsal cord, epidurally, on the side of the pain
Central lesion (dorsal spinal root, cord, brain)	Thalamic sensory nucleus, somatotopically on the side opposite to the pain
2. Ischemic	Dorsal cord, epidurally
II. Involuntary movements	
1. Dyskinesias with sensory disturbances	Ventroposterolateral thalamus (sensory nucleus), somatotopically
2. Extrapyramidal tremor – Second side (bilateral) – Speech disturbances – Psycho-organic syndrome	Ventrolateral thalamus
3. Cerebellar tremor – Second side (bilateral) – Speech disturbances – Psycho-organic syndrome	Ventrolateral thalamus

on the location of the lesion (thalamic or parathalamic) on computerized tomography[6]. The series of phantom pain and the one of neuropathic pain in the extremities comprise patients who did not experience reduction in pain with epidural dorsal cord stimulation.

The major advantages of both techniques, spinal cord and sensory thalamic neurostimulation, is the reversibility of the operation, and its non-destructive character. Neurological sequelae following the implantation of an electrode have been never observed. The two major problems with spinal cord stimulation are: 1) The migration of the electrode when using the percutaneous system, but this is very rare with the electrode implanted via a laminotomy. 2) The lead breakage (up to 14% according to the material used) which requires revision of the system. However, improvement of the material has been achieved in the last few years. Whether the dorsal cord, the dorsal spinal root or the thalamic sensory nucleus has to be stimulated depend on the location, the level and the extension of the neuropathic painful area (Table 5).

As with the implantation of foreign materials in general, we have to report up to 6% infection in both series. A few patients may develop an allergy to the material used in the system (1%). A study of the stimulation parameters on long-term shows that in the epidural cord systems, the intensity of the stimulation has to be gradually increased in the first few weeks, due probably to the formation of scar tissue at the tip of the electrode. With deep brain electrodes, the parameters of stimulation are very stable, demonstrating the safety of the method without pathophysiological modifications of the brain tissue over the years.

This long-term follow-up of a large series of patient suffering from chronic intractable pain demonstrates that the best indication for dorsal spinal cord, dorsal spinal root and sensory thalamic stimulation is pain due to direct involvement of nervous tissue (chronic neuropathic or neurogenic or deafferentation pain). Pain in ischemia is the second best indication for electrical neurostimulation; in this group, not only pain relief may be achieved, but also healing of small ischemic ulcers thanks to improvement of microcirculation (Tables 4 and 5).

II. Neurostimulation for Involuntary Movements

Since the first report of deep brain stimulation for movement disorders by Bechtereva in Leningrad in 1972[1], very few controlled studies have been published. Chronic stimulation of the subthalamic region was successfully used by Brice and McLellan in 1980[4], who reported suppression or decrease of severe intention tremor in 3 female multiple sclerosis patients. They used continuous stimulation with 75 – 150 Hz and square-wave pulses of 0.5 – 1 mA of 200–400 microsec. duration. To reduce the total amount of stimulation, the transmitter was controlled by a switching device triggered by electromyographic signals from the deltoid muscle of the appropriate arm. Sensory thalamic nuclei as target point in therapeutic stimulation for dyskinetic movements has been emphasized by Mazars[12], who reported marked improvement of involuntary movements in 17 cases of deafferentation pain of different origins, all associated with dyskinesias. In 1985 we could confirm this spectacular effect[16]. In 1987, Benabid reported his first series of Parkinsonian tremor well controlled by chronic stimulation of the nucleus V.im. of the thalamus through implanted stimulators[2]. In this volume, our experience of 19 cases of Parkinsonian tremor, 2 cases of essential tremor and 1 case of complex tremor is analysed and the value as well as the limit of the method presented[3].

Continued stimulation of thalamic structures in the treatment of involuntary movements is an attractive method and has to be considered as an alternative therapeutical approach when serious side effects of the classical high-frequency coagulation can be anticipated (for instance bilateral operations) (Table 5).

III. Neurostimulation for Spasticity

1. Dorsal Cord Stimulation

The use of electrical stimulation in the treatment of paralysed and spastic muscles is an old method and was recommended more than 100 years ago. Electrotherapy has since been widely used by physiotherapists. In 1973 Cook and Weinstein first observed amelioration of neurological dysfunction in a patient with multiple sclerosis who had a spinal cord stimulator implanted for relief of pain[5]. A significant modification of neurological disturbances was reported after prolonged observation in four additional patients with multiple slerosis: a) decrease of extensor spasticity in leg and of flexor spasticity in arm; b) progressive improvement of the synergy of movement of non-paralysed muscles; c) return of voluntary motor control in some muscles; d) lowering of the threshold for various sensory stimuli. Despite the major advance of chronic intrathecal Baclofen administration for the management of spasticity, we still consider the dorsal cord stimulation in moderate, still useful spasticity, as an attractive alternative, particularly when neuropathic pain is also present.

2. Sensory Thalamic Stimulation

In 1980, we implanted two sensory thalamic nuclei electrodes, one on each side, in a 41 year old patient suffering from deafferentation pain in the legs after traumatic paraplegia and associated with severe spasticity. There was virtually immediate control of pain and clonus with bilateral VPL stimulation. After stimulation was stopped, the clonus reappeared over two minutes. These bilateral systems were also programmed for one minute of stimulation each 2 minutes, later on each minute. An additional case has been operated since then and the same observation has been made[15]. Chronic thalamic stimulation for spasticity could be an indication when pain due to deafferentation is also present.

IV. Neurostimulation for Breathing Control

In 1959, Glenn began to apply radiofrequency stimulation to the phrenic nerve in patients with respiratory insufficiency and developed an implantable phrenic pacer[9]. In 1981, already over 295 implants have been used with about 118 in quadriplegics and the remainder in patients with syringomylia, post-cordotomy apnea, sleep apnea and spinal muscular atrophy. Long-term follow-up have shown that the best indications for electrophrenic stimulation are ventilatory insufficiency due to interruption of the upper motor neurons of the phrenic nerve and malfunction of the respiratory control centre (central hypoventilation syndrome, sleep apnea or "Ondine's curse"). In a recent review of his personal experience of thirty-five cases operated on and followed up to 10 years, Fodstad emphasizes the value of the method, but pleads for the concentration of this technique to a few centres with the adequate resources and experience[8].

V. Neurostimulation to Control Bladder Emptying

In 1970, Nashold implanted a bipolar electrode in the conus medullaris of a 17-year-old paraplegic male for emptying his bladder, and the result was over the years very good. Analysing a large series. Nashold mentions good results in 55.6% of paraplegics[14]. The indications are limited, but in some cases this method can be of real value.

Conclusions

After three decades of development and applications of therapeutic neurostimulation in functional neurosurgery with implantation of electrodes and neuropacemakers, a balanced view on its usefulness and

Table 6. *Indications which can be Considered in Neurological Disorders*

I. Spasticity Spinal origin slight to moderate	Dorsal cord, sensory thalamic nucleus
II. Chronic hypoventilation, Respiratory paralysis	Phrenic nerve
III. Bladder control	Conus medullaris

Table 7. *Disputed Indications for Chronic Therapeutic Neurostimulation in Functional Neurosurgery*

I. Pain Somatogenic (nociceptive)	Dorsal cord stimulation Periaqueductal-periventricular gray substance stimulation
II. Involuntary movements Dyskinesias	Dorsal cord stimulation (cervical) Cerebellar stimulation
III. Prolonged post-traumatic unconsciousness, vegetative state	Deep brain stimulation

limitation is possible. The best indications as well as the best targets in the nervous system to be stimulated can now be defined (Table 5). Some indications are rare, but may be considered (Table 6). Finally, more questionable indications can be mentioned (Table 7). The techniques for supplementing or replacing loss of function in neurologically impaired individuals with the implantation of neural prothesis are still experimental.

The use of implanted programmable neuropacemakers has great potential for producing significant benefits for mankind. The reversibility and the relative safety of the method are factors of particular importance. It is probable that with better definition of indications and lower cost of devices this form of treatment may be more commonly utilized over the next few years. However, the method should still be deployed on well-defined and strict indications.

References

1. Bechtereva NP, Bondartchuk AN, Smirnov VM, Meliutcheva LA (1972) Therapeutic electrostimulations of the deep brain structures. Vopr Neirkhnir 1: 7–12
2. Benamid AL, Pollak P, Louveau A, Henry S, de Rougemont J (1987) Combined (thalamotomy and stimulation) stereotactic surgery of the VIM thalamic nucleus for bilateral Parkinson disease. Appl Neurophysiol 50: 344–346
3. Blond S, Siegfried J (1991) Thalamic stimulation for the treatment of tremor and other movement disorders. Acta Neurochir (Wien) [Suppl] 52: 109–111
4. Brice J, McLellan L (1980) Suppression of intention tremor by contingent deep brain stimulation Lancet ii: 1221–1222
5. Cook AW, Weinstein SP (1973) Chronic dorsal column stimulation in multiple sclerosis. New York State J Med 73: 2868–2872
6. Demierre B, Siegfried J (1985) Le syndrome douloureux thalamique. Corrélations anatomo-cliniques et traitement par stimulation intermittente des noyaux sensitifs du thalamus. Neurochirurgie 31: 281–285
7. Devor M, Wall PD (1981) Plasticity in the spinal cord sensory map following peripheral nerve injury in rats. J Neurosci 1: 679–684
8. Fodstad H (1989) Pacing of the diaphragm to control breathing in patients with paralysis of central nervous system origin. Stereotact Funct Neurosurg 53: 209–222
9. Glenn WWZ, Hegeman JH, Mauro A (1964) Electrical stimulation of excitable tissue by radio-frequency transmission. Ann Surg 160: 338–350
10. Hood TW, Siegfried J (1984) Epidural versus thalamic stimulation for the management of brachial plexus lesion pain. Acta Neurochir (Wien) [Suppl] 33: 451–457
11. Mazars GJ, Choppy JM (1983) Reevaluation of the deafferentation pain syndrome. In: Bonica JJ *et al* (ed) Advances in pain research and therapy, Vol. 5. Raven Press, New York, pp 769–993
12. Mazars G, Merienne L, Cioloca G (1980) Control of dyskinesias due to sensory deafferentation by means of thalamic stimulation. Acta Neurochir (Wien) [Suppl] 30: 239–243
13. Meyerson BA (1990) Neuropathic pain: an overview. In: Lipton S *et al* (ed) Advances in pain research and therapy. Vol. 13, Raven Press, New York, pp 193–199
14. Nashold BS, Friedman H, Grimes J (1982) Electrical stimulation of the conus medullaris to control bladder emptying in paraplegia: a ten-year review. Appl Neurophysiol 45: 40–43
15. Shealy CM, Mortimer JT, Reswick J (1967) Electrical inhibition of pain by stimulation of the dorsal column: preliminary clinical reports. Anesth Analg 46: 489–491
16. Siegfried J (1986) Effets de la stimulation du noyau sensitif du thalamus sur les dyskinésies et la spasticité. Rev Neurol 142: 380–383
17. Siegfried J (1990) Neurostimulation techniques for intractable pain in the hand and the wrist. In: Wynn Parry (ed), Management of pain in the hand and the wrist, Churchill Livingstone, Edinburgh (in press)
18. Wall PD (1983) Alterations in the central nervous system after deafferentation: connectivity control. In: Bonica JJ, *et al* (ed), Advances in pain research and therapy, Vol. 5, Raven Press, New York, pp 679–689

Correspondence: J. Siegfried, AMI Klinik Im Park, Seestrasse 220, CH-8002 Zürich, Switzerland.

Acta Neurochirurgica, Suppl. 52, 118–120 (1991)

Epidural Spinal Electrical Stimulation in the Treatment of Severe Arterial Occlusive Disease

U. Steude[2], **D. Abendroth**[1], and **L. Sunder–Plassmann**[1]

[1] Department of Surgery, [2] Department of Neurosurgery Klinikum Grosshadern, University of Munich, Federal Republic of Germany

Summary

The effect of epidural spinal cord stimulation (ESES) on peripheral circulation in 10 cases with advanced vascular occlusive disease has been tested, using transcutaneous oxygen measurement ($TcpO_2$), contact thermography and laser-speckle measurements.

The values in all cases increased. Improvement was more pronounced during the first 2–3 weeks.

Indications and limitations of this treatment modality are discussed.

Keywords: Epidural spinal cord stimulation; peripheral circulation; vasculare occlusive disease; transcutaneous oxygen measurement; contact thermography; laser–speckle measurement.

Introduction

Due to increasing life expectancy vascular surgeons are increasingly confronted with severely threatened extremities due to an advanced peripheral arterial occlusive disease. The three existing therapeutic approaches are: surgical revascularisation, primary amputation and conservative treatment.

Unfortunately, in absence of a peripheral run off vessel, revascularisation is not effective in approximately 20% of cases and primary amputation is burdened with a high mortality[1]. For these patients unsuitable for or unsuccessfully treated by vascular surgery other therapeutic modalities should be considered. Epidural spinal cord stimulation (ESES)[2,5] which was originally aimed for the treatment of disorders such as chronic intractable pain, bladder dysfunction and multiple sclerosis, has been suggested to improve the peripheral blood supply to the limb and to reduce amputation rate[2,3,4]. Although the true mechanism of increased blood flow by ESES is not clear, there are reports discussing the decrease of sympathetic nerve activity shown by the decrease in plasma nor-epinephrin and decreased C-fibre imput[5,6].

Attempts have been made to delineate the beneficial clinical effects of ESES with the use of xenon-washout techniques, ankle pressure measurements or plethymography. All these techniques failed to evaluate the effects of ESES on microcirculation.

Material and Methods

Instead of quantitative flow measurements, non-invasive methods like the combination of transcutaneous oxygen measurement ($TcpO_2$ and telethermography as well as a new method called laser-speckle similar to the laser doppler method, measuring the red cell blood movement in the skin[7,8], are now used. $TcpO_2$ measures the dilatation reserve capacity under local hyperthermia (44°C) using a Kontron-electrode. The thermocamera indicated that only patients in advanced stage consistently showed a distal borderline of perfusion, an important area for the attachment of the $TcpO_2$-electrode.

Capillary flow is indirectly registered by the $TcpO_2$ electrode. With thermocamera, additional, semiquantitative conclusions can be drawn on thermoregulatory shunt flow behaviour, because skin surface temperature is affected by subdermal and intradermal capillary flow. Whenever changes in local skin flow are induced by any therapeutic modality it should be possible to detect and register these changes.

As part of an effort to develop a standardized non-invasive methodology to diagnose vascular diseases related primarily to the cutaneous circulation, we evaluated the postocclusive reactive hyperaemia response (reoxygenation-time) monitored by $TcpO_2$.

Laser-speckle register the red cell blood flow in the skin by utilizing the dynamic laser effect.

The indication was limited to those cases where a positive effect of sympathectomy can be expected on the basis of a positive reaction to pharmacologic sympathic blockade by peridural anaesthesia. Patients receive a peridural catheter and are tested with 10 ml bupivacain 0.5%.

The efficiency of ESES in advanced stages of arteriosclerotic disease (Fountain's stage III + IV; III n = 3 and IV n = 7) was studied in 10 patients (mean age 69.5 years) using $TcpO_2$ measurements. Contact thermography and laser-speckle measurements were used as well. The mean duration of intermittent claudication was 23.9 months and the duration of present stage, 6.7 months.

All patients had inoperable lower limb ischaemia with occluded crural arteries technically unsuitable for reconstructive surgery.

Conservative treatment or vasoactive drugs had failed. Treatment was started with an Itrel pacing system after a "test" with peridural anaesthesia. Mean follow-up period was 12 months.

An Itrel epidural electrode was inserted percutaneously to the Th12 vertebral level and epidural spinal cord stimulation was started using a pulse width of 270 microsec., a pulse rate of < 100 Hz and a mean amplitude of 7.4 volts.

The examination was performed in a temperature-controlled room with a set temperature of 23.5 ± 1.4°C. All subjects were in a comfortable supine position. Values are given as mean $\pm$ SEM. Differences were tested using the Wilcox rank test for paired samples. The difference is significant at $p<0.05$.

Results

The 2-years patient and limb survival rate, calculated by the cutler adherer formula, showed a 85% 2-year-survival for patients and 72% for the extremities (Fig. 1).

$TcpO_2$-values registered on dorsum of foot increased from 13.4 ± 3 mmHg to 34 ± 4 mmHg ($p<0.001$). There was a faster increase of values in the first 2 to 3 weeks than in the following period (Fig. 2). Telethermography showed an improved perfusion with an increase of temperature of 1.72°C ($\pm$0.36°C).

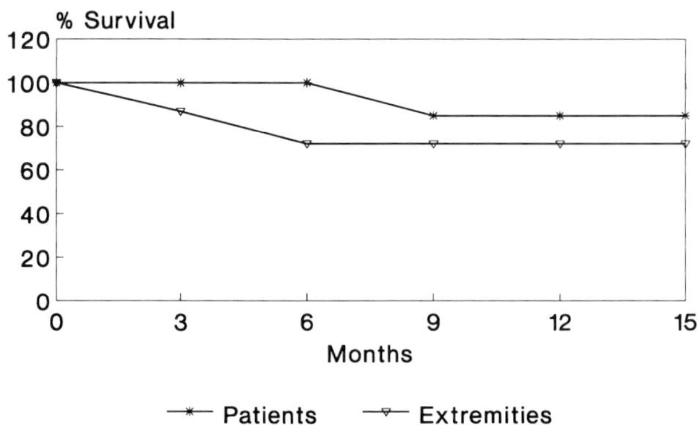

Fig. 1. 2-years patient and limb survival after ESES in Stage III +IV patients

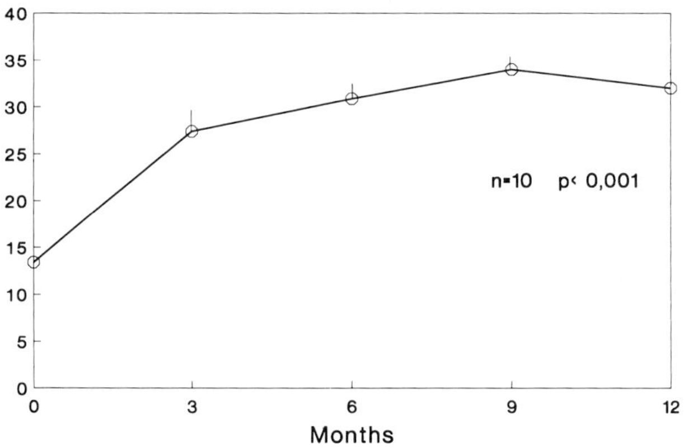

Fig. 2. Increase of TcpO2—values after ESES in Stage III +IV Patients

Laser-speckle measurement showed a significant increase of red cell blood flow from 0.26 ± 0.11 to 0.38 ± 0.16 relative units ($n = 7$).

One patient was amputated after 5 months due to an acute event. Another limb was lost after 4 months due to lack of cooperation. Cessation of pain was observed in all patients and the amount of analgesics was reduced to 15%. Phantom-pain was not developed after amputation probably due to the use of ESES.

Discussion

In arterial occlusive disease with failed conventional treatment ESES may have a beneficial effect but appears to be less suitable for the rapidly, progressive form. With reduced patient compliance, ESES should not be applied, especially after prior lumbar sympathectomy.

A beneficial effect of a continuous peridural sympathetic blockade must be evaluated from two points of view:

Besides the pain relief and improved blood supply, a "steel-phenomenon" could occur, and without the "alarm-function" of pain, there may be a critically reduced blood supply to the extremity. This could explain the poor results in use of ESES in advanced stages of arterial occlusive disease. Because of the individual variation in outcome, it is difficult to define the indications for this mode of treatment. In our hands, it is not employed unless a previous test has shown a positive effect.

Still unsolved are problems such as the cost/benefit.

Conclusion

Although our experience with ESES is relatively limited, our results suggest that in patients with an advanced stage of arterial occlusive disease ESES should be considered as an alternative treatment. The observed pain relief and possible limb salvage require further investigations. It appears that ESES should be tried only in cases with a positive effect of a sympathetic blockade. However, a clear definition of indications and mechanisms involved warrant further study.

References

1. Largiader J (1988) Therapie bei Verschluss der A. Poplitea mit und ohne Beteiligung cruraler Arterien. Operative Manahmen. In: Alexander Kriessmann (Hrsg) Aktuelle Diagnostik and

Therapie in der Angiologie. Georg Thieme Verlag, Stuttgart, New York, pp. 111–116
2. Augustinson LE, Holm J, Carlsson CA, Jivegard L (1985) Epidural electrical stimulation in severe limb ischemia: Pain relief, increased blood flow and a possible limb-saving effect. Ann Surg 202: 104–110
3. Grunkemeier GL, Starr A (1977) Actuarial analysis of surgical results: rationale and method. Ann Thorac Surg 24: 404–408
4. Fiume D (1983) Spinal cord stimulation in peripheral vascular Pain. Appl Neurophysiol 46: 290–294
5. Tallis RC, Illis LS, Sedgwick EM, Hardwidge, Gardfield JS (1983) Spinal cord stimulation in peripheral vascular disease. J Neurol Neurosurg Psychiatry 46: 478–484
6. Kaada B (1982) Vasodilatation induced by transcutaneous nerve stimulation in peripheaml ischemia. Eur Heart J 3: 303–306
7. Sunder-Plassmann L, Messmer K, Becker H M (1981) Tissue pO_2 and transcutaneous pO_2 as guidelines in experimental and clinical drug evaluation. Angiology 32: 686
8. Abendroth D, Sunder-Plassmann L, Becker HM. Use of telethermography and transcutaneous pO_2 for therapeutic control in arterial occlusive disease. In: The thoracic and cardiovascular surgeon, Vol 33, Georg Thieme Verlag, Stuttgart New York, p 25

Correspondence: U. Steude, Department of Neurosurgery, Klinikum Grosshadern, University of Munich, Federal Republic of Germany.

Acta Neurochirurgica, Suppl. 52, 121–123 (1991)

Dorsal Column Stimulation (DCS): Cost to Benefit Analysis

S. Bel and **B.L. Bauer**

Department of Neurosurgery, Philipps University of Marburg, Marburg, Federal Republic of Germany

Summary

In order to analyse the ratio of costs to clinical benefit of the implantation of a neurostimulator (type Medtronic SE-4) we examined a group of 14 patients who required treatment for chronic lumboischialgia after repeated surgery for herniated discs. Over a period of two years we evaluated the pre- and postimplantation costs. The implantation of a DC-Stimulator resulted in a striking decrease in drug requirements, in the total time of clinical treatment, and in the degree of disability. The DCS provides a satisfying method of treatment for chronic lumboischialgia after repeated surgery for herniated discs. Despite relatively high primary costs, treatment with a DCS results in a significant decrease in the accumulated expenses in comparison to other methods of medical treatment in similar cases.

Keywords: Chronic lumboischialgia; DCS; cost of implantation; drug consumption; work capacity.

Introduction

Dorsal column stimulation (DCS) or spinal cord stimulation (SCS) has proved to be an important method of alleviating pain ever since its introduction in 1967[6]. In particular, treatment of pain in chronic lumboischialgia after multiple unsuccessful intervertebral disc operations[2,10], is often the last chance for a pain ridden patient.

Since in the world at large, chronic lumboischialgia belongs to the most common causes of invalidity (in the B.R.D. it ranks third), its costs play an important role[11]. For example, in the B.R.D. around 700,000 patients per year are treated for lumboischialgia. This entails a loss of 13 million work days. In Switzerland[8] this loss has been estimated to be around 600 million Franks; in the U.S.A., the costs are around 12 billion dollars a year.

Since the percentage of patients with lumbalgia and the costs caused by this condition are so high, the question arises as to whether the costs involved with the implantation of a neurostimulator are justifiable when compared with classical pharmacological therapy[9].

Material and Methods

In the Neurosurgical Department of the University of Marburg, 14 patients (8 men, 6 women) with chronic lumboischialgia after multiple intervertebral disc operations were implanted with a DCS neurostimulator (Type: Medtronic SE-4) between the years 1987–1988.

A variety of alternative methods of treatment had failed on each patient. Lumboischialgia was the most prevalent symptom in 8 patients, bilateral ischialgia in 3 patients, unilateral ischialgia in 2 patients and lumbalgia in 1 patient. In all, 13 patients suffered from radicular pain, one from pseudoradicular pain.

Twelve patients were actively employed; two had already been retired because of chronic pain. All of the patients who were still employed had been repeatedly absent from work due to illness in previous months. The last pain-therapy has been limited to different analgesic medications. The decision to implant a DCS was taken on the following exclusion criteria:

(1) The presence of an organic (mechanical) cause for the complaint (all patients had been examined by myelography and computer tomography with intrathecal contrast medium).
(2) Opiate addiction.
(3) Evidence of psychiatric illness.
(4) TENS (Transcutaneous electrical nerve stimulation) had proven to be ineffective.
(5) DCS-induced pain-reduction of less than 30% during percutaneous trial (see below).

The implantation of the DCS was carried out in two sessions. In the first session-under local anesthesia – the electrode was percutaneously guided to its epidural target. Then, after a 7-day trial with an external neurostimulator, in the second session under local or general anesthesia – the neurostimulator-receiver was implanted subcutaneously. There were no surgical complication. Along the 2 years following implantation, electrode malfunctions were reported in a total of 7 patients. The average life span of the electrodes was 14, 2 months with an average 1, 5 electrodes per patient over two years. These factors were negative factors in the material and treatment costs. The period of Hospitalization accounted for an average of 17 days, including reoperations.

Results

Our analysis is based on the following factors:
(1) subjective judgement of pain-alleviation after DCS.
(2) costs of equipment and medications used for implantation.
(3) costs of hospitalization.
(4) length of postoperative work-disability as well as the ability to return to work.

With respect to these factors:
(1) For over 2 years, the patients were examined every 3 months. According to the effectiveness of the neurostimulation, they were divided into 5 groups.

As is evident from Fig. 1, the pain-reducing effect decreases in direct proportion to the elapsed time after the operation. At the end of the time period analyzed, the pain-reducing effect was still present in 8 of 11 patients.
(2) All these patients needed large quantities of analgesics prior to implantation. According to the type of drugs used, the patients were divided into 5 groups and their consumption of medications evaluated every 3 months.

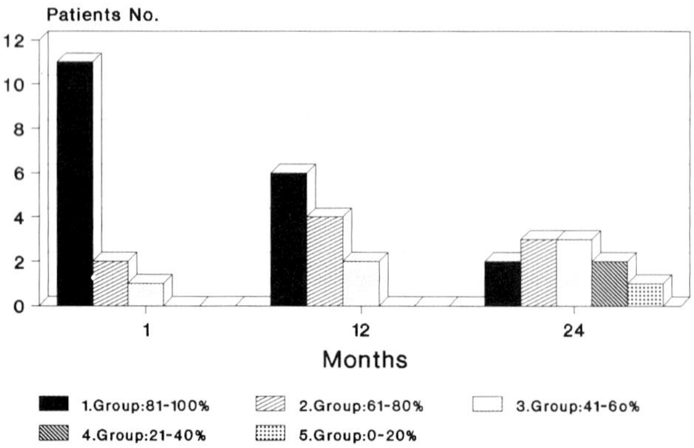

Fig. 1. Results of the DCS

As can be seen from Fig. 2, the consumption of drug's could be significantly reduced by DCS. After 2 years of DCS-therapy, 45% required no further medication. None of the other patients required pain-medication on a regular basis but only occassionally (for example after physical exertion). No patients needed strong analgesics. The average preoperative cost of medication per patient, per year was 3553.00 DM. Due to the reduction in the use of drugs after DCS (only occassional use, minimal doses), the postoperative cost for medications was drastically reduced. The average cost per patient was less than 400.00 DM per year.

In contrast to the decreased costs of medication, however, the cost of neurostimulators has consistently increased. The acquisition of a neurostimulator (Medtronic Type SE-4), including the electrode, cost 10,761.00 DM. Due to the relatively short lifetime of the electrodes, the total cost of materials came to 11,761.00 DM per patient.
(3) The time of hospitalization was an average of 17 days (including hospitalization due to electrode revision). At a daily cost of 629.00 DM, the total cost of hospitalization comes to 10,700.00 DM and the total costs for the implantation thus amount to around 22,467.00 DM.
(4) Postoperatively, all patients who had jobs were excused from work due to illness for an average of 3 weeks. Of 12 patients with jobs, 7 went back to work after the operation. Figure 3 shows the capacity to work among patients with a DCS (average back to work-quotient was 66,7%). That amounts to 39% when considering all patients originally with jobs, over the total time period of 288 months.

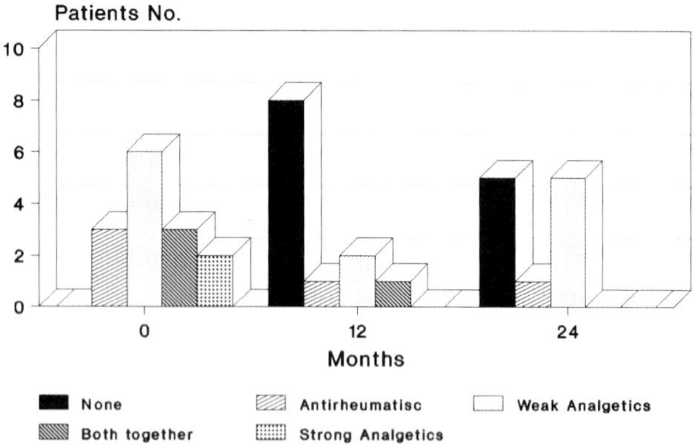

Fig. 2. Classification according to type of pharmaceutical

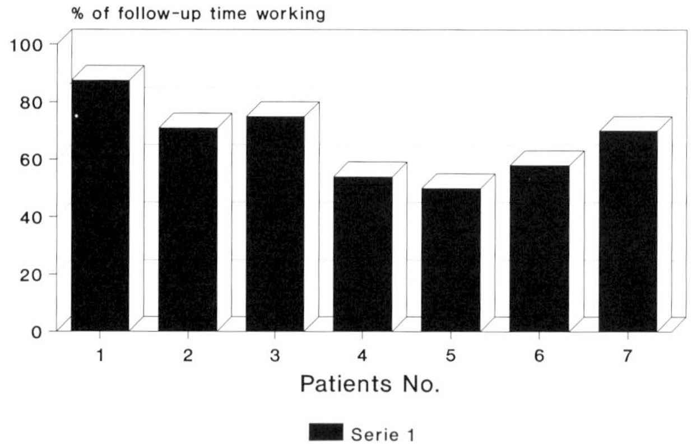

Fig. 3. Post-operative work capacity

Discussion

Pain therapy with DCS brought significant pain relief to all patients. The high costs of acquisition and electrode replacement were partially compensated for by the drastic reduction of pharmaceutical expenses (Fig.2). Furthermore, the postoperative work-capacity of the patients was significantly increased (Fig.3)

Thus, the primary high expense for the DCS was quickly recovered by the renewed earning power generated by the patients reentrance into the work-world and the reduction of pharmaceutical costs.

DCS has proven to be a justifiable means of cost reduction, in patients with chronic lumboischialgia after repeated unsuccessful intervertebral disc operations.

References

1. Davis R, Gray E (1981) Technical factors important to dorsal column stimulation. Appl Neurophysiol 44: 160–170
2. Demirel T, Braun W, Reimes CD (1984) Results of spinal cord stimulation in patients suffering from chronic pain a two year observation period. Neurochirurgia 27: 47–50
3. Dimitrijevic MR, Faganet J, Sherwood AM (1983) Spinal cord stimulation as a tool for physiological research. Appl Neurophysiol 46: 245–253
4. Erikseo DL, Long DM (1983) Ten years follow-up of dorsal column stimulation. In Bonica JJ *et al* (eds) Advances in pain research and therapy. Vol 5, Raven Press, New York, pp 583–590
5. Halter J, Dolenc V, Dimitrijevic MR, Sharkey PC (1983) Neurophysiological assessment of electrode placement in the spinal cord. Appl Neurophysiol 46: 124–128
6. Nashold BS, Friedman H (1972) Dorsal column stimulation for control of pain. J Neurosurg 36: 590–597
7. Nielson KD, Adams JE, Hosobuchi Y (1975) Experience with dorsal column stimulation for relief of chronic intractable pain. Surg Neurol 4: 148–152
8. de La Porte Ch, Siegfried J (1983) Lumbosacral spinal fibrosis (spinal arachnoiditis). Its diagnosis and treatment by spinal cord stimulation. Spine 8: 593–603
9. Richardson R, Signeira E, Cerullo L (1979) Spinal epidural neurostimulation for treatment of acute and chronic intractable pain: initial and long term results. Neurosurgery 5(3): 344–348
10. Shatin D, Mullet K, Hults G (1986) Totally implantable spinal cord stimulation for chronic pain: disain and efficiency. PACE 9: 577–583
11. Zimmermann M (1975) Neurophysiological models for nociception, pain and pain trerapy. Springer, Berlin Heidelberg New York Tokyo. Adv Neurosurg 3: 199–225

Correspondence: S. Bel, Department of Neurosurgery, Philipps University of Marburg, Marburg, Federal Republic of Germany.

Pain

Acta Neurochirurgica, Suppl. 52, 127–129 (1991)

Does Microsurgical Vascular Decompression for Trigeminal Neuralgia Work Through a Neo-Compressive Mechanism?

Anatomical-Surgical Evidence for a Decompressive Effect

M. Sindou, F. Amrani, and **P. Mertens**

Department of Neurosurgery and UFR Grange Blanche, Hopital Neurologique et Neurochirurgical Pierre Wertheimer, University of Lyon, Lyon, France

Summary

The positive effect of Microsurgical Vascular Decompression (MVD) on idiopathic trigeminal neuralgia[3,4] still remains controversial between a decompressive mechanism and a "neo-compressive" one[1].

This paper is a summary of a comparative study of the results on pain obtained with two technical modifications of the MVD procedure. The first consisted of interposition of a foreign material between the nerve and the transposed artery after dissection of the trigeminal nerve, whilst in the second the offending vessel(s) was dislodged without using any material touching the nerve.

The two series of 60 patients in each were similar concerning the clinical features. Evaluation of results on neuralgia – with one year follow-up-in both series, shows that the technique used in the second group was not followed by a higher rate of recurrence than the technique used in the first group. On the contrary; 4.5% in the 2nd group compared to 10% in the first.

This indicates that MVD would not act as a result of "neo-compression" of the nerve, but rather through a real decompressive mechanism.

Keywords: Microsurgical vascular decompression; neurovascular conflict; trigeminal nerve; trigeminal neuralgia.

Material and Methods

From 1986 to date, freeing the nerve from its vascular compression was performed with maximum precautions so as not to touch it even slightly. The offending vessel (s) was dislodged apart by means of small strings of Teflon (2 mm in width, 4 cm in length)[2], and when necessary a rectangular piece of Dacron (7×10 mm) supported by the superior petrosal vein, but without contact with the nerve, was used[5] (Fig. 2). From our total series of MVD of more than 400 cases (1974–1988), for this study we have selected two groups with 60 patients in each. The first group (1984–1986) corresponds to the last 60 patients who underwent the "old" procedure (Fig. 1). The second group (1986–1988) was the first 60

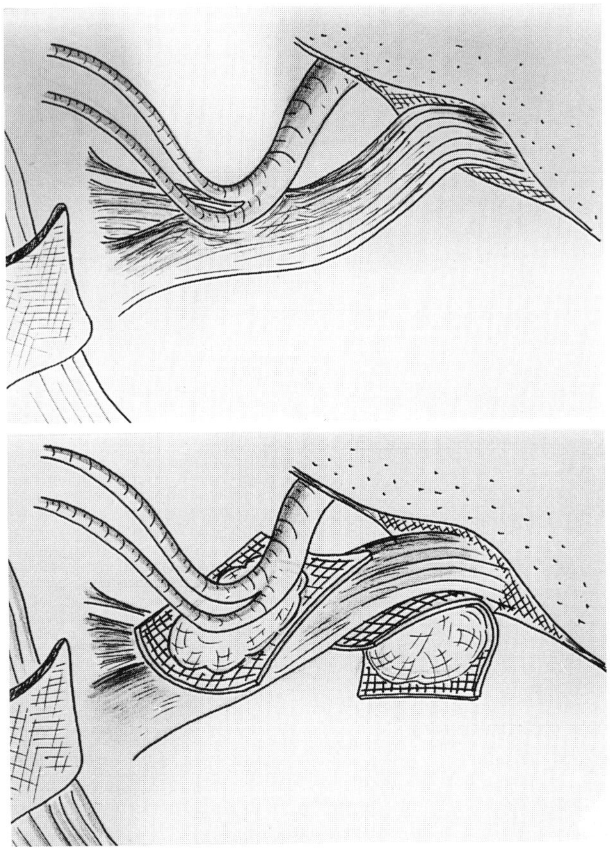

Fig. 1. Decompression with interposition
Top: neurovascular conflict depressing the right Vth root entry zone by superior cerebellar artery, associated with nerve angulation when crossing the petrous ridge
Bottom: microvascular decompression and restitution of the normal course of the nerve, using Dacron and periosteum

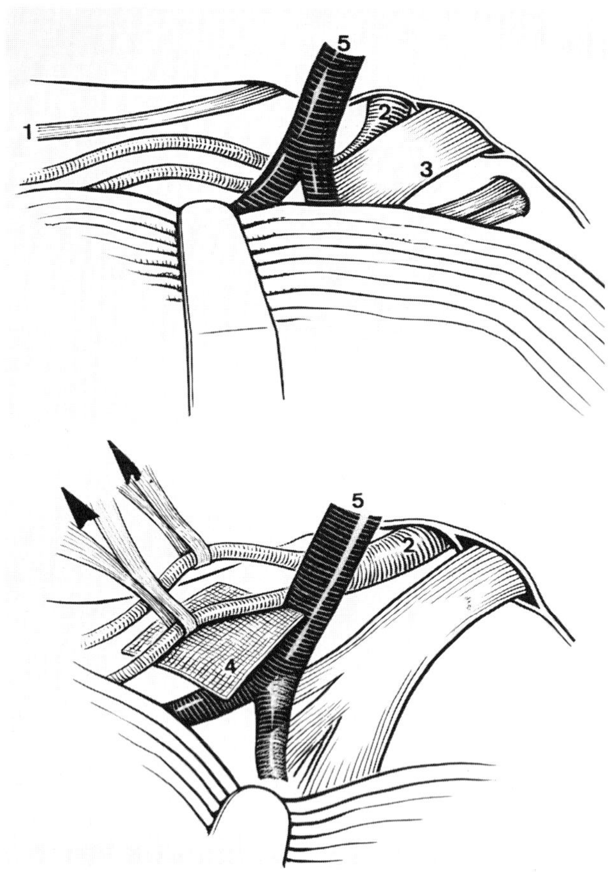

Fig. 2. Decompression without interposition
Top: After retraction of the supero-lateral aspect of the right cerebellar hemisphere (with preservation of the superior petrosal vein (5), the dorso-lateral part of the peripedoncular cistern along the trochlear nerve (1) is opened, so as to release the superior cerebellar artery (2) which compresses the trigeminal nerve (3)
Bottom: Docompression of the trigeminal nerve by transposition of the superior cerebellar artery (2) without interposition of material. The two branches of the artery are maintained apart by two strings of Teflon (arrows) flattened along the inferior wall of the tentorium cerebelli and a piece of Dacron (4) supported by the superior petrosal vein (5)

Table 1. *Types of Neuro-Vascular Conflicts*

	SCA	SCA + AICA	SCA + VEIN	SCA + AICA + VEIN	VEIN	NO NVC; Arachnoid adhesions
Group I	39	6	9	1	2	3
Group II	29	14	12	0	2	3
Total (120 Cases)	68	20	21	1	4	6

patients operated on with the "atraumatic – non compressive" method. Both groups were similar with regard to sex, age, clinical features, and anatomical findings at operation (Table 1).

Result on Pain

This paper aims to compare the results on pain only. Detailed descriptions of complications and side-effects of both techniques have been given elsewhere[5]. Table 2 shows the immediate post-operative results, and Table 3 the long-term results. Pain was completely relieved, without hypesthesia and/or dysesthesia, in 75% in group I (mean follow-up: 41 months) and in 83. 3% in group II (mean follow-up: 16 months). Evaluation of the results after one year in both series (Fig. 3) showed that the technique used in the second group was not followed by a higher rate of recurrence than the technique used in the first group. On the contrary, there was 4.5% recurrence in the second group compared to 10% in the first group.

Table 2. *Immediate Post-Operative Results*

	Total Cure	Partial Cure	Failure
Group I	42 (70%)	17 (28, 3%)	1 (1, 7%)
Group II	51 (85%)	9 (15%)	0
Total (120 Cases)	93 (77, 6%)	26 (21, 6%)	1 (0, 8%)

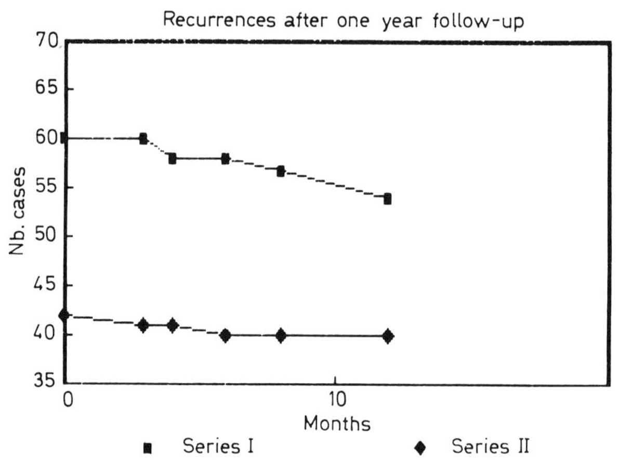

Fig. 3. Actuarial curve of patients pain-free, along the first year of follow-up, in both series

Table 3. *Long-Term Post-Operative Results*
(Mean follow-up: Group I: 41 months; Group II: 16 months)

	Total Cure	Partial Cure	Recurrence
Group I	45 (75%)	7 (11,7%)	8 (13, 3%)
Group II	50 (83, 3%)	8 (13, 4%)	2 (3, 3%)
Total (120 Cases)	95 (79, 2%)	15 (12, 5%)	10 (8, 3%)

Discussion and Conclusion

A larger number of patients and a longer period of follow-up are of course needed before definitive conclusions concerning the mechanism of cure after MVD[1,3,4] can be drawn. Although the atraumatic nature of the technique used in the second group was only relative, we want to stress that there was a significant difference between the two technical modalities. During the second procedure no material touching the nerve was interposed. However, it can be argued that a secondary and delayed arachnoiditis may have a role in the long-term pain relief. Nevertheless, in our opinion, the results in this preliminary study indicate that MVD does not act by a "neocompression" of the nerve, but by a real decompressive mechanism.

References

1. Adams CBT (1989) Microvascular compression, an alternative view and hypothesis. J Neurosurg 70: 1–2
2. Fukushima T (1986) Personal communication
3 Gardner WJ (1962) Concerning the mechanism of trigeminal neuralgia and hemifacial spasm. J Neurosurg 19: 947–958
4 Jannetta PJ (1967) Arterial compression of the trigeminal nerve at the pons in patients with trigeminal neuralgia. J Neurosurg 26: 159–162
5 Sindou M, Amrani F, Mertens P (1990) Decompression vasculaire microchirurgicale pour névralgie du trijumeau, Neurochirurgie 36: 16–26

Correspondence: M. Sindou, Hopital Neurologique, 59 Bd Pinel, F-60003 Lyon, France.

Acta Neurochirurgica, Suppl. 52, 130–132 (1991)

Neurones with Epileptiform Discharge in the Central Nervous System and Chronic Pain

Experimental and Clinical Investigations

K. Yamashiro[1], **K. Iwayama**[1], **M. Kurihara**[1], **K. Mori**[1], **M. Niwa**[1], **R.R. Tasker**[2], and **D. Albe-Fessard**[3]

[1]Department of Neurosurgery and Second Department of Pharmacology, Nagasaki University School of Medicine, Nagasaki, Japan, [2]Department of Neurosurgery, Toronto General Hospital, University of Toronto, Toronto, Canada and [3]Department of Physiology, I.N.R.A. Jouy en Josas, France

Summary

Epileptiform discharge was recorded from neurons in the thalamic nuclei of chronic pain patients during stereotactic surgery. Hyperactive neurons showed regular firing of 3–5 trains of epileptic-like group discharges with a frequency of 4 to 5 Hz.

As described by Lombard *et al.* (1979), we operated on the dorsal root unilaterally, sectioning C5 to Thl in male Wistar rats. One to three months after the operation, hyperactive neurons were examined in the contra-lateral thalamic nuclei (VP, zona incerta), and lemniscus medialis.

The firing patterns and distribution of hyperactive neurons in these animals was very similar to those of humans. The hyperactive neuron was unaffected by electrical stimulation of the nucleus raphe dorsalis (NRD) and locus ceruleus (LC). Administration of phenytoin and diazepam reduced the firing. However, no effect was seen with valproic acid. During spreading depression of the sensorimotor cortex, a remarkable reduction was seen on the firing of thalamic hyperactive neurons. This suggested that hyperactive neurons of the thalamic nuclei received facilitory effects from the sensorimotor cortex with little influence from adrenergic or serotoenergic systems.

Keywords: Chronic pain; epileptic-like hyperactive neuron Denervation; spreading depression.

Introduction

Loeser *et al.*[8] and Tasker *et al.*[11] have reported epileptic-like discharges from (hyperactive) neurons in the spinal posterior horn and in thalamic nuclei in patients with chronic pain. Also, it has been reported that after injury to sensory nerves in the periphery, epileptic-like discharge from hyperactive neurons were observed at the posterior horn, brain stem, thalamus and cerebral cortex in experimental animals[1,2,7,9]. The purpose of this paper is to examine the hyperactive neurons with epileptiform discharges, which were recorded from chronic pain patients and in thalamic nuclei of denervated rats.

Material and Methods

Eight chronic pain patients were examined. Causes of pain were peripheral nerve injury in two, spinal cord injury in two, in one each with stump pain, trigeminal neuralgia, cerebrovascular disease and multiple sclerosis. Prior to implantation of chronic stimulating electrodes for the treatment of pain, extracellular unitary recording and local microstimulation were performed in the ventral caudal (Vc) nucleus of thalamus using the same microelectrode[11].

In animal experiments, unilateral dorsal roots sectioning from C5 to Thl in male Wistar rats were made according to the method and chronic pain model of Lombard *et al.*[9]. After unilateral dorsal root sectioning, contralateral thalamic units, ECoG and DC potentials of sensorimotor cortex were recorded. The effects of locus ceruleus (LC) and nucleus raphe dorsalis (NRD) stimulation, and sensorimotor cortical spreading depression[6] on cellular behaviour were examined. The effect of phenytoin, diazepam and valproic acid on the unitary discharge was also investigated. Specific binding sites for substance P in denervated rats were examined using an autoradiographic method with 125 I-Bolton-Hunter substance P [10].

Results

Clinical Results

Epileptiform discharges (from hyperactive neurones) were recorded from the thalamus of chronic pain patients (Fig. 1). Two types of firing pattern were seen. One showed regular firing which had 3–5 trains of epileptiform grouped discharges with a frequency of 4 to 5 Hz (middle and lower trace in Fig. 1). The

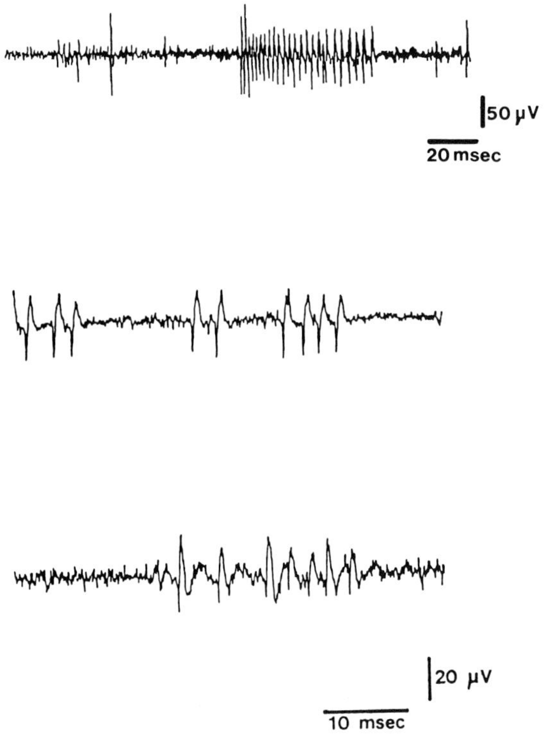

Fig. 1. Epileptic-like discharge (hyperactive) neurons from the human thalamic nuclei. Upper trace shows continuous firing. Middle and lower trace shows multiple train firing pattern

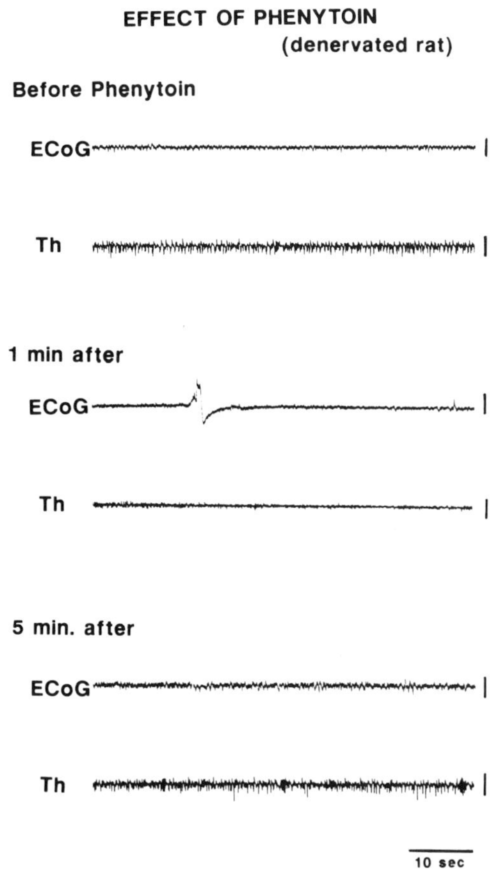

Fig. 2. Effect of phenytoin. One minute after drug administration, the thalamic hyperactive neurons were remarkably suppressed but recovered 5 minutes after administration. Electrocorticogram (ECoG) was also affected

other showed continuous firing, as shown in upper panel of Fig. 1. These hyperactive neurons were distributed in ventrocaudal (Vc), ventral intermediate (Vim), ventral oral posterior (Vop) nuclei of thalamus. Most of them were seen in a place 14mm lateral to the midline.

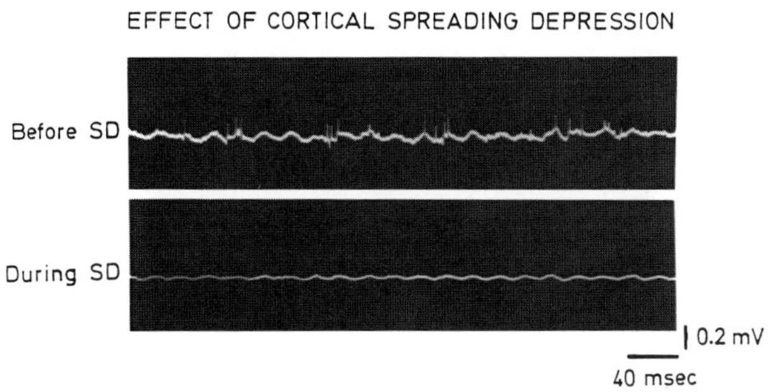

Fig. 3. Effect of cortical spreading depression (SD) on thalamic hyperactive neurons. Before SD (upper trace), 3 to 4 trains of a hyperactive neuron was seen. During SD (lower trace), the hyperactivity was suppressed

Experimental Results

After sectioning of the cervical dorsal root, the rat showed self-mutilation of the right forepaw, or shoulder area. The basal ganglia and thalamus of the denervated side showed slight reduction of substance P binding sites. One to three months after the operation, epileptiform discharges from hyperactive neurons were recorded from the thalamic nuclei (VP, zona incerta), lemniscus medialis and internal capsule. The electrical stimulation of LC and NRD showed little effect on the firing pattern of hyperactive neurons. Administration of valproic acid had no effect on the firing of hyperactive neurons. Diazepam showed a small decrease in thalamic neuronal firing. However, one minute after administration of phenytoin, thalamic hyperactive unit firing showed remarkable reduction, which then recovered (Fig. 2).

The effect of cortical spreading depression (SD) on thalamic hyperactive neurons is showed in Fig 3. During cortical spreading depression, hyperactive neurons showed remarkable reduction in firing.

Discussion

After sensory tract injury at the peripheral or spinal cord level, intermittent multiple firing neurons have been found in the posterior horn, brain stem, thalamus and cortex in experimental animals[1,2,7,9]. Loeser *et al.* and Tasker *et al.* recorded epileptiform discharges from hyperactive neurons in injured human spinal cord and thalamic nuclei[8,11]. Loeser outlined a correlation between epileptiform neuronal discharges and pain[8]. The firing patterns of human hyperactive neurons and those of animals in our results were very similar to those reported earlier. The anti-epileptic drugs showed different effects on the hyperactive neurons. Although Defeudis reported that GABAergic agonists induce analgesia[3], valproic acid and a GABAergic agonist, did not affect the hyperactive neurons. Diazepam showed a slight decrease and phenytoin a marked decrease in firing. The effect on neurons descending from the cortex to the spinal posterior horn has been reported as both facilitatory and inhibitory[1,4]. From our results, we conclude that thalamic hyperactive neurons received a facilitatory effect from sensorimotor cortex. Recently, Katayama *et al.*[5] reported that electrical stimulation of human motor cortex reduced the pain. This suggests that suppression of cortical function reduces the firing of hyperactive neurons.

References

1. Albe-Fessard D, Lombard MD (1983) Use of an animal model to the origin of and projection against deafferentation pain. In: Bonica JJ, Lindblom U, Iggo U (eds) Advances in pain research and therapy, Vol 5, Raven Press, New York, pp 691–700
2. Anderson LS, Black RG, Abraham J, Ward AA Jr (1972) Neuronal hyperactivity in experimental trigeminal deafferentation. J Neurosurg 35: 444–452
3. Defeudis FV (1982) GABAergic analgesia: naloxone intensive system. Pharmacol Res Commun 14: 383–390
4. Giuffrida R, Sanderson P, Condes-Lara M, Albe-Fessard D (1986) Corticofugal influences on dorsal column nuclei: an electrophysiological study in the rat using the cortical spreading depression technique. Exp Brain Res 61: 649–653
5. Katayama Y, Tsubokawa T, Maejima S *et al* (1989) Brain stimulation for the treatment of intractable pain: Stimulation of thalamic sensory relay nucleus and motor cortex. Funct Neurosurg 28: 67–72
6. Leao AAP (1944) Spreading depression of activity in the cerebral cortex. J Neurophysiol 7: 359–390
7. Loeser JD, Ward AA Jr (1967) Some effects of deafferentation on neurons of the cat spinal cord. Arch Neurol 17: 629–636
8. Loeser JD, Ward AA Jr, White LE Jf (1968) Chronic deafferentation of human spinal cord neurons. J Neurosurg 29: 48–50
9. Lombard MC, Nashold BS, Pelissier T (1979) Thalamic recordings in rats with hyperalgesia. In: Bonica JJ, Lindblom U, Iggo A (eds) Advances in pain research and therapy, Vol 3, Raven Press, New York, pp 767–772
10. Niwa, M, Shigematsu K, Plunkeatt L, Saavedra JM (1985) High-affinity substance P binding sites in rat sympathetic ganglia. Am J Physiol 249: H694–H697
11. Tasker RR, Lenz FA, Yamashiro K *et al* (1987) Microelectrode techniques in localization of stereotactic targets. Neurol Res 9: 105–112

Correspondence: K. Yamashiro, Department of Neurosurgery Nagasaki University School of Medicine, 7–1 Sakamotomachi, Nagasaki, 852 Japan.

Acta Neurochirurgica, Suppl. 52, 133–136 (1991)

Pathophysiology of Central (Thalamic) Pain: A Possible Role of the Intralaminar Nuclei in Superficial Pain

M. Hirato, Y. Kawashima, T. Shibazaki, T. Shibasaki, and **C. Ohye**

Department of Neurosurgery, Gunma University, Gunma, Japan

Summary

In 15 patients with central pain (thalamic pain) after stroke, CT, PET scan and intraoperative thalamic microrecordings were performed. The results are considered together to evaluate a possible role of thalamic intralaminar nuclei in the genesis of central pain, especially of superficial pain.

In the non-thalamic lesion group (deep pain dominant), thalamic background neural activity (BNA) was relatively high in Vim but low in CL. Conversely, in the thalamic lesion group (superficial pain dominant), thalamic BNA was higher in CL than in Vim, and markedly decreased in VC. In this group, regional cerebral oxygen consumption (rCMRO2) was relatively maintained, and regional oxygen extraction ratio (raOEF) and the relative value of regional cerebral glucose utilization (CMRGL), compared to rCMRO2, was increased in the cerebral cortex around the central sulcus. The genesis of superficial pain is discussed.

Keywords: Superficial pain; thalamic intralaminar nuclei; depth microrecording; PET Scan.

Introduction

We have previously presented results related to the pathophysiology of the deep pain component in central pain states based on findings on CT, PET scan and intraoperative thalamic microrecordings. These results indicate that deep pain is associated with functional changes in the thalamic Vim nucleus after a partial destruction of the VC nucleus[3].

In this paper we discuss the possible role of intralaminar nuclei for the genesis of central pain, especially of the superficial pain component.

Patients and Methods (Table 1)

Stereotactic Vim-CL thalamotomy was carried out in 6 cases, Vim thalamotomy in 2 cases, and Vim-Vcpc thalamotomy in 7 cases. According to CT findings, they were classified in two groups: (A) non-thalamic lesion group including cases with apparently normal CT and (B) thalamic lesion group. Clinical features of central pain were classified as deep pain and superficial pain. It was noticed that deep pain was more marked in cases in which the CT scan revealed no definite thalamic damage, and superficial pain in cases with definite thalamic damage.

At stereotactic thalamotomy, microrecording was made using Leksell's stereotactic apparatus[4]. Sequential background neural activity and unitary and multiunitary spike discharges were analyzed by quantitative estimation of amplitude averaging method, and by power averaging method (PAV) (sampling time 0.5 msec, bandpass between 7 Hz and 1000 Hz, averaging 30 times) separated by frequency band. Observations were made in conscious patients under local anaesthesia.

PET studies were performed in 11 cases of central pain and 5 control cases, using a steady-state method with C15O2–15O2[2]. 18FDG studies were also performed in 3 cases of central pain with Sokoloff's method[5]. In our PET laboratory, the CT and the PET scanners are installed in parallel, and a single-patient-bed slides between them. Thus, the centres of each slice in CT and PET are adjusted automatically, making precise comparisons possible. Regional blood flow, rOEF, rCMRO2 and CMRGL in central pain patients were measured in the thalamus, caudate nucleus, putamen, globus pallidus, and cerebral cortex. Averaged rCMRO2 were compared in both central pain and control groups. Oxygen-glucose molar utilization ratios (OGMUR) were also calculated.

Results

A. Electrophysiological Study of Thalamus in Patients with Central Pain

In Parkinsonian patients (control), the PAV histogram was relatively homogeneous in and around the Vim nucleus, the profile of which displayed one peak configuration between O Hz and 800 Hz with a maximum at 100–200 Hz. In the non-thalamic lesion group of central pain, the PAV histogram showed a slight reduction with a mixture of various activities in and around the Vim nucleus, and multiple peak configurations between O Hz and 1000 Hz with a

Table 1. *A list of the Operated Patients*

CENTRAL PAIN

No	Case	Lesion	Stroke	Sensory disturbance	Op.	BNA(VIM)	(CL)	PET
				A. Thalamic lesion (-)				
a.lesion (-)								
1	N.K. 49 m	(L)	inf	D++, S+, H', (bp), pst	Vim-CL	+	+	
2	T.T. 46 m	(L)	inf	S++, (bp)	Vim-CL	+	+	
b.Putaminal lesion								
1	J.H. 52 m	L	hem	D++, S+, H',	Vim-CL	+	+	
2	T.T. 48 f	R	inf	D++, S+, H', dst	Vim-CL	+	+	●
3	K.K. 60 m	L	hem	S++, H',	Vim-(Cd)	+		●
4	G.M. 64 m	L	hem	D++, S+, H', (bp)	Vim	+		●
5	S.K. 66 f	L	hem	S++, H',	Vim-Vcpc	+		●
6	M.A. 76 m	L	hem	D+, S+, H',	Vim-Vcpc	+		●
7	H.T. 54 f	R	hem	D++, S+, H', (dst)	Vim-Vcpc	+		●▲
8	M.T. 53 m	L	hem	D++, S+, H', (dst)	Vim-Vcpc	+		●▲
				B. Thalamic lesion (+)				
1	M.N. 61 m	L	hem	D+, S++, H',	Vim-CL	+	+	
2	K.S. 69 f	R	inf	D+, S++, H',	Vim-CL	+	+	●
3	T.Y. 54 m	R	inf	S++, H', (bp), dst	Vim-Vcpc	+		●
4	K.I. 54 m	L	hem	S++, dst	Vim-Vcpc	+		●
5	K.S. 43 f	R	inf	S++, H', dst	Vim-Vcpc	+		●▲

D:deep pain (movement related) S:superficial pain (with numbness) inf:infarct
H':hyperpathia pst:paresthesia dst:dysesthesia bp:burning pain hem:hemorrhage
●: PET – GAS(rCMRO2) ▲: FDG(rCMRGlu) BNA:background neural activity

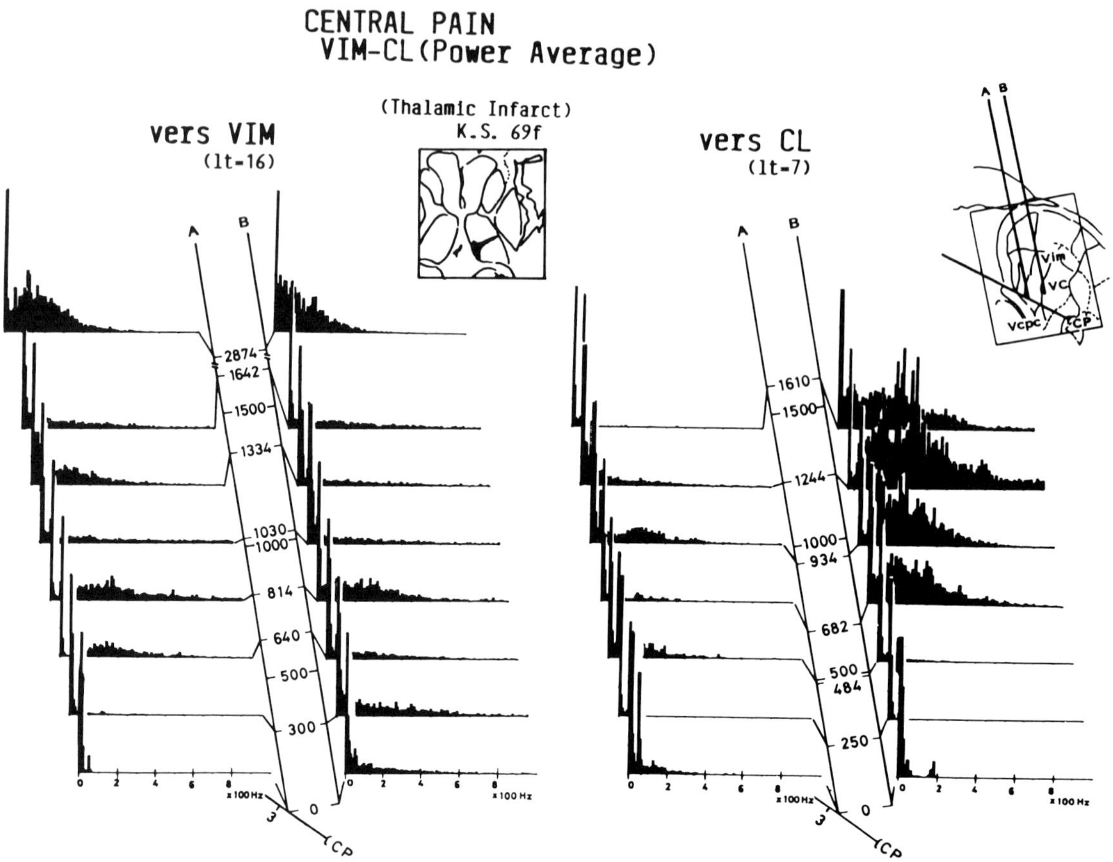

Fig. 1. Profiles of neural activity in and around Vim nucleus and in intralaminar nuclei (CL) in a thalamic lesion case of central pain, estimated by power averaging method (PAV). Upper middle figure shows location and size of the thalamic lesion. Upper right figure shows the relationship between trajectories A and B and the thalamic subnucleus. In the PAV histograms, distance readings from the target point are shown in 10 μm unit, and transverse axis shows frequency between 0 Hz and 1000 Hz

maximum at 200–300 Hz. Thalamic BNA in and around Vim was comparable to that of Parkinsonian patients. BNA in intralaminar nuclei (CL) was generally low. In the thalamic lesion group of central pain, however, the PAV histogram showed marked decrease in and around the Vim nucleus. BNA in CL was higher than in Vim, especially in its dorsal part (Fig. 1). BNA in CL in this group was also higher than in the non-thalamic lesion group. The PAV histogram in CL showed higher peak frequency of between 200 Hz and 400 Hz. In case T.T., without any CT lesion but a dominant superficial pain, it is noteworthy that BNA in Vim was low, while, BNA in CL was relatively high.

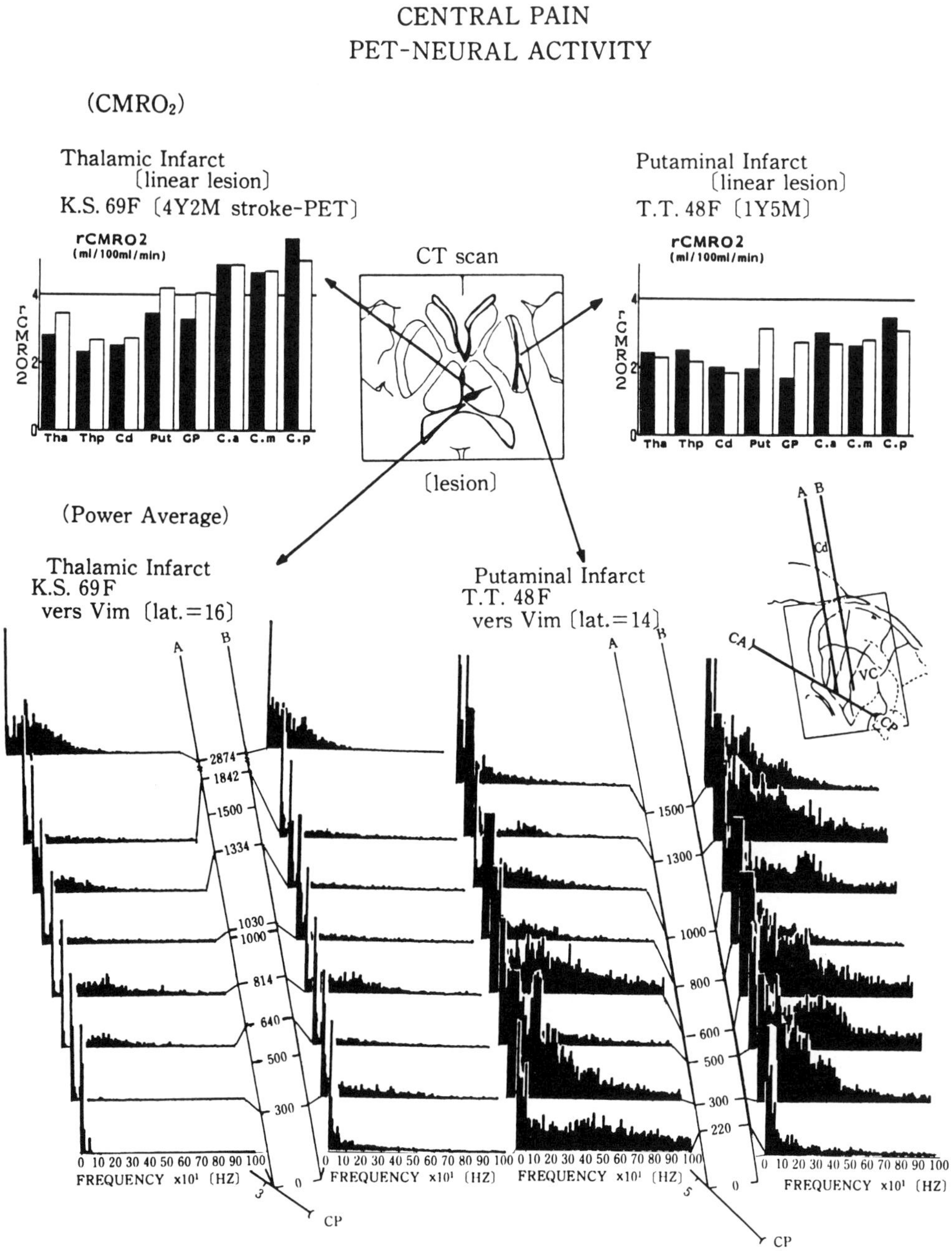

Fig. 2. Correlation between neural activity in and around Vim nucleus and regional cerebral metabolism. Middle figure in upper column shows the location and size of the cerebrovascular lesion in each case shown on CT scan. Upper left figure shows regional cerebral oxygen consumption (r$CMRO_2$) and bottom left thalamic neural activity estimated by the power averaging method (PAV) in a thalamic lesion case. Upper right shows r$CMRO_2$ and bottom right PAV in a putaminal (non-thalamic) lesion case. In the PAV histograms, distance readings from the target are shown in $10\,\mu m$ unit. From left to right in each graph of r$CMRO_2$, paired bar graphs show r$CMRO_2$ of thalamus, caudate nucleus, globus pallidus, and cerebral cortex. The filled bars represent values obtained from the side of the lesion

B. Metabolic Study by PET scan

In the thalamic lesion group with pain, rCMRO2 was relatively well maintained in most brain structures except on the lesioned thalamus. In the cerebral cortex around the central sulcus, the rCMRO2 level was almost normal. Furthermore, rOEF was also increased in that region. In the putaminal lesion group with pain and in the thalamic lesion group without pain, however, rCMRO2 was reduced in all brain structures, as was also rOEF (Fig. 2). In a thalamic lesion case with pain, glucose metabolism of the cerebral cortex around the central sulcus was also maintained, whereas OGMUR was decreased, showing an increased relative value of CMRGL compared to rCMRO2 in this structure. In a putaminal lesion case with pain, glucose metabolism was also decreased as rCMRO2, wheareas OGMUR increased in each brain structure examined.

Discussion

Electrophysiological study of the thalamus in thalamic lesion patients with central pain showed that BNA (background neural activity) was markedly decreased in and around Vim nucleus, suggesting a damage in specific sensory relay nuclei. BNA in CL was, however, higher than in Vim, and was also higher than those in CL in the non-thalamic lesion group. It should be noted that BNA in thalamic intralaminar nuclei was maintained in the thalamic lesion group. The metabolic study by PET scan in this group showed that rCMRO2 was relatively well maintained in the cerebral cortex around the central sulcus. This suggests that the function of nonspecific activating afferences, including the thalamic intralaminar nuclei, was maintained[1]. Moreover, increased rOEF and decreased OGMUR (relative value of CMRGL compared to rCMRO2) in the cerebral cortex around the central sulcus in this group may be a reflection of thalamocortical activity. Based on the electrophysiological and metabolic studies, it is suggested that the different clinical features of central pain (superficial and deep) are associated with different local pathophysiology in the thalamus.

References

1. Baron JC, D'antona R, Pantano P *et al* (1986) Effects of thalamic stroke on energy metabolism of the cerebral cortex. A positron tomography study in man. Brain 109: 1243–1259
2. Frackowiak RSJ, Lenzi GL, Jones T, Heather JD (1980) Quantitative measurement of regional cerebral blood flow and oxygen metabolism in man using 15O and positron emission tomography: Theory, procedure, and normal values. J Comput Assist Tomogr 4: 727–736
3. Hirato M, Kawashima Y, Shibazaki T, Ohye C (1989) Stereotactic thalamotomy: Pathophysiology of deep pain and superficial pain. Acta Neurochir (Wien) 98: 104–105
4. Hirato M (1990) Pathophysiology of thalamic pain. 2. Electrophysiological characteristics of thalamus in patients with thalamic pain. Kitakanto Igaku 40: 521–539 (in Japanese)
5. Sokoloff L, Reivich M, Kennedy C *et al* (1977) The (14C)-deoxyglucose method for the measurement of local cerebral glucose utilization: Theory, procedure, and normal values in the conscious and anaesthetized albino rat. J Neurochem 28: 897–916

Correspondence: M.Hirato, Department of Neurosurgery, Gunma University, 3–39–15, Showamachi, Maebashi, Gunma, 371, Japan.

Acta Neurochirurgica, Suppl. 52, 137–139 (1991)

Chronic Motor Cortex Stimulation for the Treatment of Central Pain

T. Tsubokawa, Y. Katayama, T. Yamamoto, T. Hirayama, and **S. Koyama**

Department of Neurological Surgery, Nihon University School of Medicine, Tokyo, Japan

Summary

Twelve patients with deafferentation pain secondary to central nervous system lesions were subjected to chronic motor cortex stimulation. The motor cortex was mapped as carefully as possible and the electrode was placed in the region where muscle twitch of painful area can be observed with the lowest threshold. 5 of the 12 patients reported complete absence of previous pain with intermittent stimulation at 1 year following the initiation of this therapy. Improvements in hemiparesis was also observed in most of these patients. The pain of these patients was typically barbiturate-sensitive and morphine-resistant. Another 3 patients had some degree of residual pain but considerable reduction of pain was still obtained by stimulation. Thus, 8 of the 12 patients (67%) had continued effect of this therapy after 1 year. In 3 patients, revisions of the electrode placement were needed because stimulation became incapable of inducing muscle twitch even with higher stimulation intensity. The effect of stimulation on pain and capability of producing muscle twitch disappeared simultaneously in these cases and the effect reappeared after the revisions, indicating that appropriate stimulation of the motor cortex is definitely necessary for obtaining satisfactory pain control in these patients. None of the patients subjected to this therapy developed neither observable nor electroencephalographic seizure activity.

Keywords: Brain stimulation; motor cortex; central pain; thalamic pain; pain.

Introduction

Any forms of therapies, including chronic deep brain stimulation, provide satisfactory pain control in only one third of cases with deafferentation pain secondary to central nervous system (CNS) lesions. Analysis of our experience with deep brain stimulation has indicated that the best effect of thalamic stimulation was frequently obtained in deafferentation pain secondary to peripheral nervous system (PNS) lesions[2,3]. In contrast, the effect of thalamic stimulation is often unsatisfactory for controlling deafferentation pain secondary to CNS lesions[2,3].

In order of develop more effective treatment for deafferentation pain secondary to CNS lesions, we have been exploring the effects of stimulation of various brain regions on such a pain for the last several years. We recently recognized that stimulation of the motor cortex can provide often excellent pain control in this group of patients. This clinical finding is in harmony with our experimental observation that thalamic hyperactivity following transection of the spinothalamic tract can be efficiently inhibited by stimulation of the motor cortex[1]. We summarize here the results obtained in a series of 12 patients treated by chronic epidural stimulation of the motor cortex.

Patients and Methods

Patient Population

A total of 12 patients were treated by stimulation of the motor cortex (Table 1). Among these patients, 6 had either a small thalamic infarct or thalamic hemorrhage, 3 had a small lesion in the posterior limb of the capsula interna caused by a putaminal hemorrhage, and the remaining 3 had either a pontine hemorrhage, multiple sclerosis or postrhizotomy pain. Intervals following the onset of the original disease to the occurrence of pain were 1–4 years. The patients had been treated by various kinds of medication (anticonvulsants and/or antidepressants). All but 2 cases displayed hemiparesis of varying degrees. The patients and their families gave informed consent for the procedures described below to be carried out.

Pharmacological Characterization

Pain in each patient, was characterized by responses to stepwise administration of thiopental and morphine (i.v., barbiturate and morphine tests). Changes in pain level was evaluated by each patient on standardized visual analog scale (VAS).

Surgical Procedures

The location of the motor cortex was estimated by bony landmarks with conventional method. Under local anesthesia, paramedian skin incision was made 1–4 cm lateral to the midline

Table 1. *Clinical data and the Effect of Motor Cortex Stimulation*

Case no.	Age/Sex	Original disease	Parmacological characteristics of pain: Barbiturate test	Morphine test	Result[a]
1	72/M	putaminal hemorrhage	sensitive	non-sensitive	excellent
2	54/M	thalamic infarct	sensitive	non-sensitive	excellent
3	62/M	thalamic hemorrhage	sensitive	non-sensitive	excellent
4	53/F	thalamic hemorrhage	sensitive	non-sensitive	excellent
5	52/M	thalamic infarct	sensitive?	non-sensitive	excellent
6	66/F	putaminal hemorrhage	sensitive	non-sensitive	excellent
7	59/F	thalamic infarct	sensitive?	non-sensitive	good
8	58/F	thalamic infarct	non-sensitive	non-sensitive	good
9	53/M	pontine hemorrhage	sensitive?	non-sensitive	good
10	55/F	putaminal hemorrhage	sensitive?	sensitive?	fair
11	42/F	multiple sclerosis	unclear	sensitive?	poor
12	48/F	postrhizotomy pain	sensitive?	non-sensitive	poor

[a]Excellent, 100% reduction; good, 80–60% reduction, fair, 60–40% reduction, poor, less than 40% reduction of pain on visual analog scale.

and contralateral to the painful area. The trephination was then placed over the estimated area of the motor cortex. An electrode array having 4 plate electrode (diameter, 0.5 cm) each separated by 1 cm (M 3587, Medtronic Co.) was inserted into the epidural space. The locations of the sensory and motor cortices were confirmed from phase reversal of the N_{20}wave of somatosensory evoked potential recorded from the electrode. When the electrode was moved from the sensory cortex to the motor cortex, the N_{20} wave turned to positive. The location of the motor cortex was again confirmed by motor evoked potential recoded in response to stimulation with the electrode. The motor cortex was mapped as carefully as possible and the electrode was placed in the region where muscle twitch of painful area could be observed at the lowest threshold.

The stimulation system was internalized after a period of 1 week of test stimulation. During this period, the effects of stimulation with different parameters were examined. Electroencephalograms were repeatedly recorded at predetermined interval.

Stimulation Procedures

Stimulations were usually applied for 5–10 min. for each time and no stimulations were given at night. The frequency and intensity were usually adjusted to 50–120Hz and the level slightly lower than the threshold for muscle twitch of painful area (less than 1 mA with 0.1–0.5 ms pulse). The effects of chronic stimulation of the motor cortex was evaluated at predetermined interval after the initiation of this therapy. Each patient was asked to express pain levels by VAS. The effect of chronic stimulation of the motor cortex was classified into 4 categories; excellent, complete disappearance of pain; good, reduction of pain level for 80–100%; fair, reduction of pain level for 40–60%; and poor, reduction of pain level less than 40%.

Results

In 10 of the 12 patients, satisfactory pain control was obtained during the initial 1 month after the initiation of this therapy. Pain subsided within a few minutes after the onset of stimulation and this effect continued for 3–6 hours following 5–10 min. stimulation. Usually, stimulation for 5–7 times a day was necessary during this earlier period.

Five of the 12 patients reported complete absence of previous pain with intermittent stimulation at 1 year following the initiation of this therapy (Table 1). During this later period, these patients stimulated for 2–3 times a day. Interestingly, improvements in hemiparesis was also observed in most of these cases. The pain of these patients was typically barbiturate-sensitive and morphine-resistant. Another 3 patients had some degree of residual pain but considerable reduction of pain was still obtained by stimulation. Thus, 8 of the 12 patients (67%) had continued effect of this therapy after 1 year.

Three patients did not respond favourably to this therapy. These patients tended to show different characteristic pharmacologically as well as neurologically in their pain. Their pain was questionable sensitive to barbiturate or morphine, or both. It appeared that abnormal severe pain evoked by movements of extremities is not responsive to this therapy. Conclusions, however, await further experience.

In 3 patients, revisions of the electrode placement were needed because stimulation became incapable of inducing muscle twitch even with higher stimulation intensity. Either epidural granulation or dislocation of the electrode was the cause of this change in 2 cases, and disconnection in one case. The effect of stimulation

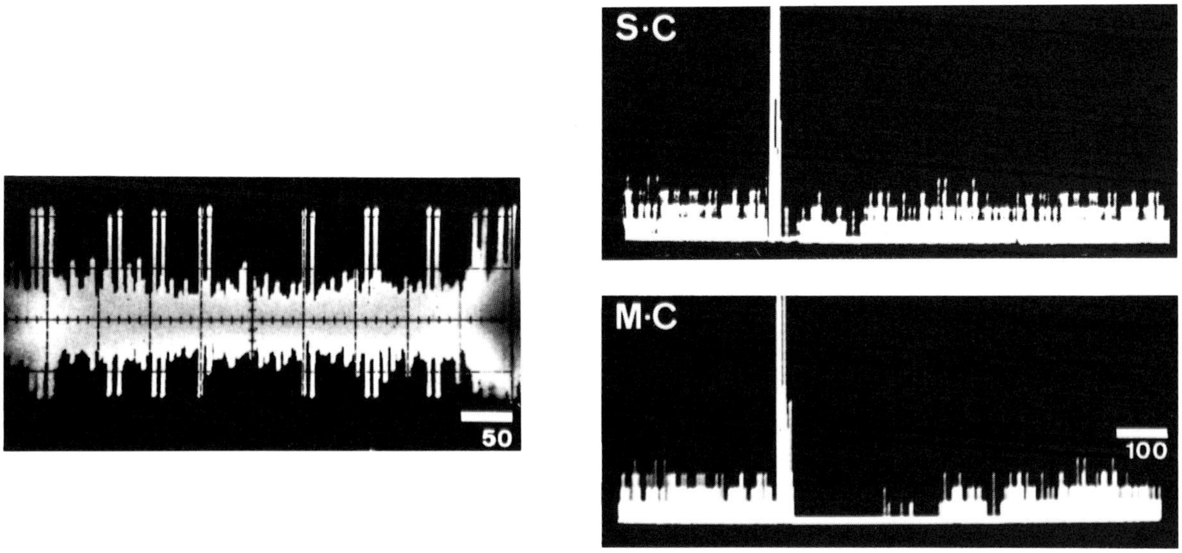

Fig. 1. A representative example of inhibitory effects of sensory and motor cortex stimulation on hyperactive thalamic neuron in the cat. Recording from thalamic relay neuron (low threshold mechanoreceptive neuron) at 3 weeks following spinothalamic tractotomy. S.C, sensory cortex stimulation; M.C, motor cortex stimulation. scales, ms

of pain and capability of producing muscle twitch disappeared simultaneously in these cases and the effect reappeared after the revisions, indicating that appropriate stimulation of the motor cortex is definitely necessary for obtaining satisfactory pain control in these patients. Stable stimulation with the technique employed in the present series of patients, which involves epidural placement of the electrode, was difficult to achieve in one patient who demonstrated moderately dilated subarachnoid space over the cerebral cortex. None of the patients subjected to this therapy developed neither observable not electroencephalographic seizure activity.

Discussion

Deafferentation pain secondary to CNS lesions is the most difficult pain to control even after the advent of chronic deep brain stimulation therapy[2,3]. Thalamic stimulation was not useful for controlling these pain. Even if the initial effect is satisfactory, tolerance to stimulation frequently develops within 7 months. In contrast, chronic stimulation of the motor cortex appears to provide better control of such pain. It also appears that the effect of stimulation of the motor cortex continues longer.

Thalamic hyperactivity is observed following experimental transection of the spinothalamic tract in cats[1]. Such hyperactivity can be inhibited more efficiently by stimulation of the motor cortex rather than sensory cortex (Fig. 1). It may be that motor cortex afferents and/or efferents activated orthodromically or antidromically can inhibit abnormal hyperactivity within the CNS underlying deafferentation pain.

The result of the present study indicates that deafferentation pain secondary to CNS lesions is better controlled by stimulation of the motor cortex rather than thalamic stimulation. It is suggested that there may be a certain subgroup of patients which respond more favourably to this therapy. The effect of stimulation of the motor cortex on hemiparesis also appears to be worthy of further studies.

References

1. Hirayama T, Tsubokawa T, Katayama Y, Yamamoto Y, Koyama S (1990) Chronic changes in activity of thalamic relay neurons following spinothalamic tractotomy in cat. Effects of motor cortex stimulation. Pain 5 [Suppl]: 273
2. Tsubokawa T (1985) Chronic stimulation of deep brain structures for treatment of chronic pain. In: Tasker RR (ed) Neurosurgery state of arts review, Vol 2. Stereotaxic Surgery, Hanley and Belfus Inc., Philadelphia, pp 253–255
3. Tsubokawa T, Katayama Y, Yamamoto T, Hirayama T (1985) Deafferentation pain and stimulation of thalamic sensory relay nucleus. Appl Neurophysiol 48: 166–171

Correspondence: T. Tsubokawa, Department of Neurological Surgery, Nihon University School of Medicine, Tokyo 173, Japan.

Acta Neurochirurgica, Suppl. 52, 140–142 (1991)

Location of a DBS-Electrode in Lateral Thalamus for Deafferentation Pain. An Autopsy Case Report

R. Kuroda, J. Nakatani, Y. Yamada, A. Yorimae, and **M. Kitano**

Department of Neurosurgery, Kinki University School of Medicine, Osaka, Japan

Summary

Pain relief was obtainable when deep brain stimulation was tried in the sensory thalamic nucleus in a patient with deaffereantation pain to cervical myelopathy. The electrode was histologically verified in post-mortem examination after 20 months and the localization of contact points of the implanted electrode was estimated. The cathode appeared to have been placed in the region from Vim to the rostral border of Vci while the anode was in the medial lemniscus region. Stimulation of the Vim nucleus might have had a pain relieving effects because no facial paraesthesiae was evoked by stimulation. The implanted electrode caused only minor histological changes.

Keywords: Pain; deep brain stimulation; thalamus.

Introduction

There have been almost no reports on histological examination on localization of electrodes implanted in the sensory thalamus in treatment of deafferentation pain by deep brain stimulation (DBS)[4] in spite of the need to confirm histologically the electrode site. We were allowed to perform an autopsy on one patient, in whom pain relief was obtained, in order to examine the localization of an electrode implanted in the brain, correlating retrospectively the stimulating sites to its effects.

Case Report

A 72-old-male, who was admitted to our hospital in 1984 because of bilateral differentiation pain, especially in the left hand and the upper extremities, due to cervical myelopathy. With dorsal column stimulation, he had enjoyed pain relief for about 7 months but eventually the effect failed. In 1987, a DBS electrode with four contact points (Medtronic) was implanted at the target of the border zone (height: −2; laterality: 13; ant to Cp: 10 mm) between the right Vce (N. ventrocaudalis externus) and the Vci (N. vetrocaudalis internus). Postoperative test stimulations was performed to determine an optimal coupling of a pair of the four contacts points. Pain relief was obtained for 9 months with a gradual decrease and minor side effects until the patient suffered from respiratory disorder due to the tuberculous pleuritis. In 1989, he died of respiratory failure. The electrode had thus been implanted for a period of 20 months.

Material and Methods

After fixation and celloidin embedding, the thalamus at the side of electrode implantation was serially cut in coronal sections (50 μm) perpendicular to the intercommissural line. Every four sections was processed with Klüver-Barrera, Holzer, HE and GFAP staining. The localization of the electrode track was assessed with reference to Hassler's classification[2]. Four contact points on the electrode were estimated by calculation, taking into account tissue shrinkage due to the fixation and celloidin embedding (20%)[7].

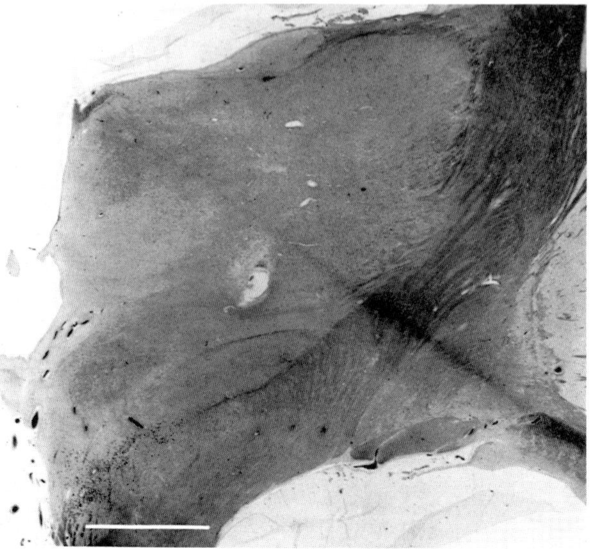

Fig. 1. Microphotograph of a representative thalamic section (section number 36, Klüver-Barrera staining, 50 μm showing an asymmetric light halo in the surroundings of the tissue defect region due to the implanted electrode. A white scale bar measures 5 mm

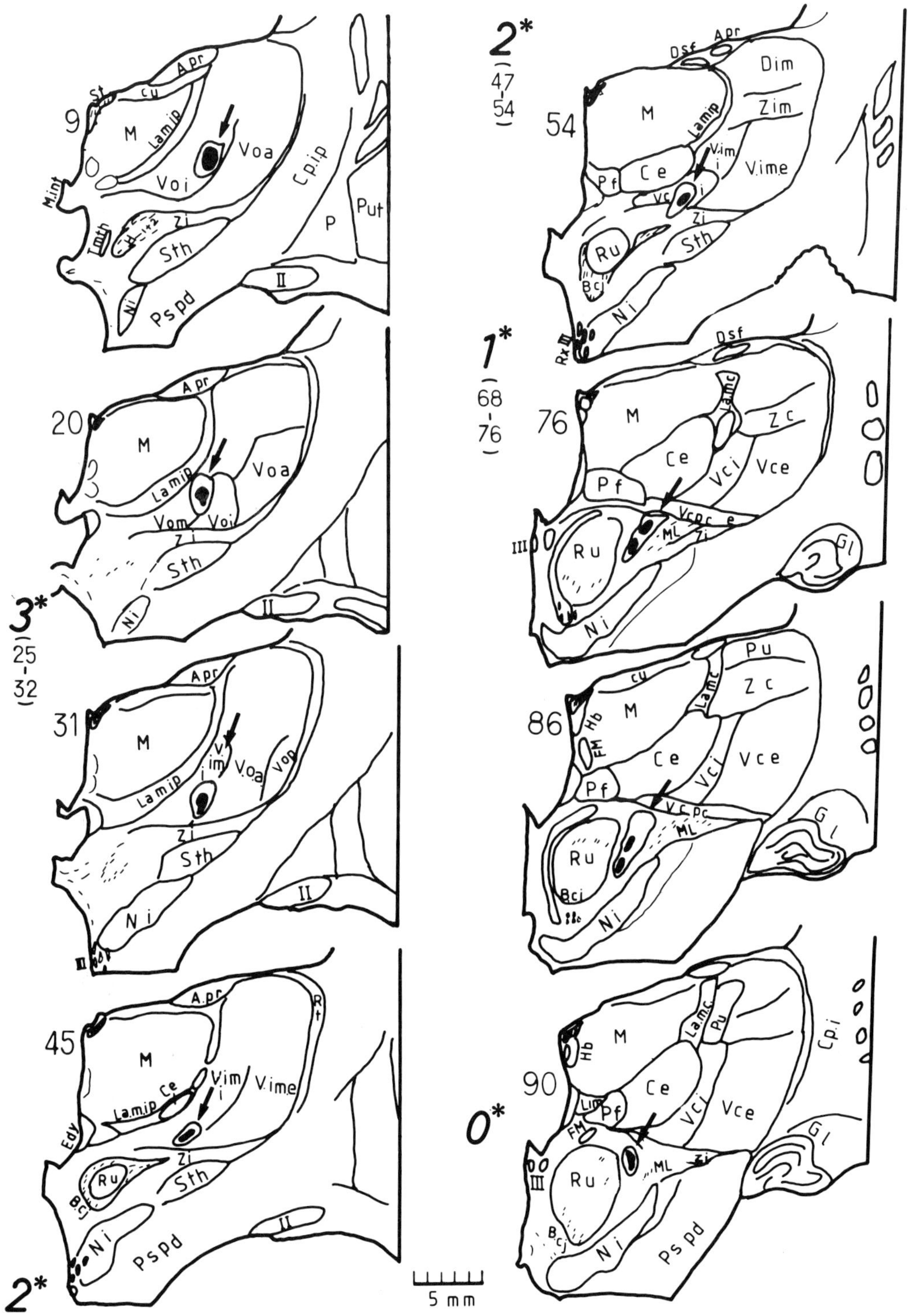

Fig. 2. Drawing of serial coronal sections indicating the electrode track (arrow) at each thalamic level. A solid black shows a defect region and its surrounding circle a light halo. Each electrode contact point at 0–3 with an asterisk (*) was indicated to the left in each figure. Numericals in parenthesis show the limit of section numbers within which the contact point was estimated to localize. Thin numericals to the left of each figure indicate the section number. Relevant abbreviations are as follows: Ce: Nucleus(N.) Centrum medianum; Lam: Lamella medialis; M: Territorium mediale thalami; ML: medial leminiscus; Pf: N. parafascicularis; Ru: Ruber; Vce and Vci: N. ventrocaudalis externus and internus respectively; Vcpc: N. ventrocaudalis parvocellularis; Vime and Vimi: N. ventrointermedius externus and internus; Voa, Voi, and Vom: N. ventrooralis anterior, internus and medialis, respectively

Results

As shown in Fig. 1 an asymmetric light halo-like zone surrounded the defect caused by the electrode, extending laterally about 200 μm and medially, as well as dorsally, about 1 mm. The myelinated fibres in the halo-zone had lost their stainability, the surroundings of the defect were encapsulated with a thin capsule, and granulation and glial proliferation extended towards the periphery of the halo zone.

As shown in Fig. 2 the electrode track appeared more medial and rostral than intended. The location of the four contact points was estimated: Point 0: medial lemniscus (ML); point 1: ML region; point 2: region of the Vimi (N. Ventrointermedius internus) and the rostral border of the Vci; point 3: region of the Vom (N. ventrooralis medialis) and the Vimi. Postoperative stimulation tests with coupling of each pair of contract points provoked paraesthesiae in the left hand, upper extremities and trunk. The couplings, having favourable effects by stimulation, were 1(−) 0(+), 1(−)2(+), 2(−)3(+) and 3(−)2(+). However, each of the pairs having good effects except 2(−)1(+), also provoked increased pain and discomfort if the strength of stimulation was increased. Oral dyskinesia was observed to disappear with stimulation in the pair 3(−)2(+). The patient complained of visual side effects with flickering sensation and pulsating sensation in the eye during stimulation. Finally, we chose the pair of 2(−)1(+) (cathode: Vimi-Vci region; anode: ML region) as the permanent coupling and implanted the receiver.

Discussion

The histological changes such as granulation and gliosis after chronic implantation of electrodes were observed within 200 μm, which is in accordance with findings of Boivie and Meyerson[1]. Histological changes (1 mm) extending medially presumably resulted from the injury caused by the medially inserted guide probe.

Contrary to our intention to stimulate the medial part of Vce nucleus, the electrode trajectory was unexpectedly verified to be localized more medially and rostrally, although one may claim that at large the target had been hit. However, the fact that the patient reported a favourable effect of stimulation for several months, it is reasonable to assume that there was a true suppression of pain. As no facial paraesthesiae were induced by stimulation, the cathode was presumably sited mainly in the Vim nucleus including part of the Vci nucleus corresponding to the contact point No 2. However, the amount of shrinkage may have been overestimated and there may also have been uncoiling of the contact points during the implantation of the electrode[3]. The patient complained of increased pain or discomfort when applying high intensity stimulation or when the polarity of the coupling was reversed: Vimi (cathode) and Vom (anode). Thus, the pain relieving effect may partly be due to anodal current activating the ML region. Interestingly, Ohye and Narabayashi[5] reported that human Vim cells react to kinesthetic deep sensation and that weak stimulation produce paraesthetic sensations although their electrode trajectory was shown to lie more laterally. It may be suggested the coupling used, cathode: Vimi (depolarization) and anode: ML (hyperpolarization), can produce somatosensory modulation. Mechanisms of pain relief with DBS, however, remains to be understood. The side effects related to vision may be due to activation of the vestibulo-thalamic fibres ascending in the vicinity, since such medullated fibres are easily excitable by electrical stimulation[6].

References

1. Boivie J, Meyerson BA (1982) A correlative anatomical and clinical study of pain supression by deep brain stimulation. Pain 13: 113–126
2. Hassler R (1959) Anatomy of the thalamus. In: Schaltenbrand G, Bailey F (eds) Introduction to stereotaxis with an atlas of the human brain. Vol 1, Georg Thieme, Stuttgart, pp 230–290
3. Hosobuchi Y (1982) Analgesia induced by brain stimulation with chronically implanted electrodes. In: Schmidek HH, Sweet WH (eds) Operative neurosurgical techniques. Indications, methods, and results. Vol 2, Grune & Stratton, New York, pp 981–991
4. Hosobuchi Y (1986) Subcortical electrical stimulation for control of intractable pain in humans. Report of 122 cases (1970–1984). J Neurosurg 64: 543–553
5. Ohye C, Narabayashi H (1979) Physiological study of presumed ventralis intermedius neurons in the human thalamus. J Neurosurg 50: 290–297
6. Ranck JBJr (1975) Which elements are excited in electrical stimulation of mammalian central nervous system: A review. Brain Res 98: 417–440
7. Van Buren JM, Borke RC (1972) Variations and connections of the human thalamus. The nuclei and cerebral connections of human thalamus. Springer, Berlin, pp 38–39

Correspondence: R. Kuroda, Department of Neurosurgery, Kinki University, 377-2, Ohno-Higashi, Osaka-Sayama, Osaka 589, Japan.

Acta Neurochirurgica, Suppl. 52, 143–145 (1991)

Bilateral Versus Unilateral Percutaneous High Cervical Cordotomy as a Surgical Method of Pain Relief

K. Amano, H. Kawamura, T. Tanikawa, H. Kawabatake, H. Iseki, Y. Iwata, and **T. Taira**

Department of Neurosurgery, Neurological Institute, Tokyo Women's Medical College, Tokyo, Japan

Summary

The present report is concerned with the results of bilateral percutaneous high cervical cordotomy (60 patients) compared with those of unilateral cordotomy (161 patients). The result of pain releif is classified into 4 grades based on Hitchcock's criteria; grade 1: complete pain relief, grade 2: almost complete pain relief with slight residual pain, grade 3: persisting pain, but tolerable, grade 4: persisting pain, untolerable. In cases of bilateral cordotomy (60 patients), 76% of the cases showed grade 1, 19% being grade 2, 3% being grade 3 and 2% being grade 4. On the contrary, the unilateral cordotomy (161 patients) showed less impressive results, particularly in grade 1, namely, grade 1 being 64%, grade 2 being 18%, grade 3 being 14% and grade 4 being 4%. Clinically acceptable results (grade 1 plus grade 2) were, therefore, obtained in bilateral cordotomy (95%) as compared with unilateral cordotomy (82%). The difference in pain relief between bilateral and unilateral procedure observed in the present investigation is contrary to that reported previously by others. The possible explanation for less impressive result in regard to grade 1 of unilateral cordotomy is that unilateral cordotomy was performed in this series to alleviate the major side of patient's pain, followed by latent pain on the other side postoperatively, which is not uncommon phenomenon in cancer pain. Whereas all of the bilateral cordotomies were done either for midline pain or bilateral pain, unilateral cordotomy gave satisfactory pain relief in some cases of midline pain. Midline pain, therefore, does not necessarily require bilateral cordotomies from a clinical point of view. Bilateral cordotomies showed good relief of pain for diffuse visceral pain, namely, 15 out of 60 patients (25%), as well as for somatic pain. Four patients (6.7%) had urinary retention more than 1 week postoperatively. There was no respiratory complication.

Keywords: Percutaneous cordotomy; unilateral; bilateral; results.

Introduction

Since 1972, 281 percutaneous high cervical cordotomies have been performed on 221 patients with intractable pain: unilateral cordotomy on 161 patients and bilateral cordotomy on 60 patients. All of these cordotomies were done with a bipolar concentric electrode. Usually percutaneous cervical cordotomy is performed with conventional monopolar electrode of Mullan type. That monopolar electrode, however, produces substantial artifact at the time of electrical stimulation, not only stimulating the lateral spinothalamic tract, but also the stimulating current extending to the nearby structures of the spinal cord, such as the pyramidal tract. It is needless to say that bipolar stimulation is preferable to monopolar stimulation for localized electrical stimulation from neurophysiological point of view. The authors devised a bipolar concentric electrode of 0.5 mm outer diameter with interpolar distance of 0.5 mm, total length of the electrode being 130 mm. This bipolar concentric electrode of small diameter has not only contributed to more precise intramedullary stimulation for analysis of the lateral spinothalamic tract in man, as previously published elsewhere[1,3,5], but markedly reduced the incidence of postoperative complications of percutaneous cervical cordotomies. The authors report the clinical results of percutaneous cordotomy using this type of electrode with special reference to bilateral procedures in comparison with unilateral procedures.

Material and Methods

Sixty patients (40 males and 20 females) had bilateral cordotomies, whereas 161 patients (92 males and 69 females) had unilateral cordotomies. Incidence of bilateral cordotomy in a total of 221 patients was 27%. The patient's age was in the range of 14 to 80 years. The result of pain relief was classified into 4 grades based on Hitchcock's criteria (Table 1). Ninety percent (198 patients) had pain due to malignancy and 10% (23 patients) had non-cancer pain of various origin. All of 60 patients with bilateral cordotomy

Table 1. *Criteria for Evaluation of Pain Relief after Cordotomy*

Grade 1:	Complete pain relief
Grade 2:	Almost complete pain relief with slight residual pain
Grade 3:	Persisting pain, but tolerable
Grade 4:	Persisting pain, untolerable

Table 2. *281 Percutaneous High Cervical Cordotomies for 221 Patients*

Bilateral Cordotomy	60 patients Male 40: Female 20	27%
Unilateral Cordotomy	161 patients Male 92: Female 69	73%

Table 3. *60 Patients of Bilateral Cordotomies*

Midline Pain	16 patients	27%
Bilateral Pain	44 patients	73%
Visceral Pain	15 patients	25%
Somatic Pain	45 patients	75%

Table 4. *Pain Relief obtained by Percutaneous Cordotomy*

	Grade 1	Grade 2	Grade 3	Grade 4
Bilateral Cordotomy (60 patients)	76%	19%	3%	2%
Unilateral Cordotomy (161 patients)	64%	18%	14%	4%
All Cases (221 patients)	67%	19%	11%	3%

had pain secondary to malignancy. Bilateral cordotomies were done for 16 patients (15 males and 1 female) of midline pain (27%) and 44 patients (25 males and 19 females) of bilateral pain (73%). All of the cordotomies were performed with bipolar concentric electrode of small diameter as described elsewhere[1] (Table 2,3).

Results

The result of pain relief is summarized in Table 4. Grade 1 – pain relief was obtained in 76% of bilateral cordotomies versus in 64% of unilateral cordotomies and in 67% of all cases. There was no difference in grade 2 – pain relief between bilateral and unilateral cordotomies. Clinically acceptable pain relief (grade 1 plus grade 2) was obtained, therefore, in 95% of bilateral cordotomies versus in 82% of unilateral cordotomies. Urinary retention of more than one week duration was seen in 4 out of 60 patients of bilateral cordotomies. Urinary retention of more than one week duration was seen in 4 out of 60 patients of bilateral cordotomy (6.7%). There was no postoperative respiratory dysfunction or neurological deficit such as motor weakness.

Discussion

Percutaneous cordotomy has provided not only good relief of pain for patients with malignant neoplasm but also elucidated the important mechanism underlying the neurophysiological function of the spinal cord of man[1,2,3,5,6]. The present report is concerned with the clinical result of pain relief, particularly the difference in pain relief between bilateral and unilateral procedures. Our results show better relief of pain in bilateral cordotomies than in unilateral cordotomies, which is contrary to the report by other investigators[4,7]. The possible explanation for less impressive result in regard to grade 1 of unilateral cordotomy is that unilateral cordotomy was performed in this series to alleviate the major side of patient's pain, followed by recognition of latent pain on the other side postoperatively, which is not an uncommon phenomenon in cancer pain. Whereas all of the bilateral cordotomies were done either for midline pain (27%) or bilateral pain (73%), unilateral cordotomy gave satisfactory pain relief in some cases of midline pain. Midline pain, therefore, does not necessarily require bilateral cordotomies. Bilateral cordotomies showed good relief of pain for diffuse visceral pain, namely 15 out of 60 patients (25%), as well as for somatic pain. Seven to ten days interval between the first and the second cordotomy gives less postoperative complications together with the use of bipolar concentric electrode of small diameter for precise intramedullary spinal cord stimulation. The follow-up period of pain relief was variable, simply because of the fact that the 90% of the patients had pain due to malignancy in advanced stage with a short life expectancy; some died within one week after cordotomy and most patients seldom survived more than three months postoperatively. In this series of patients, postcordotomy dysesthesia was, therefore, rarely encountered.

Cancer pain has two aspects, both denervation pain and non-denervation pain. The former type of chronic pain have clinical signs of denervation characterized by hypesthesia in the painful region. The latter type of more or less acute pain is due to direct stimulation by tumour mass invading peripheral nerves just like a dental drill touching the tooth pulp. In view of the fact that cordotomy has been known to be ineffective for denervation pain such as thalamic pain and that cordotomy is very effective for cancer pain, the major part of cancer pain, at least investigated in the present study, is composed of non-denervation pain.

References

1. Amano K, Iseki H, Notani M, Kawabatake H, Tanikawa T, Miyazaki T, Kawamura H (1979) Percutaneous cordotomy and cerebral evoked response. Appl Neurophysiol 42: 316
2. Hitchcock E, Leece B (1967) Somatotopic representation of the respiratory pathways in the cervical cord of man. J Neurosurg 27: 320–329
3. Iseki H, Amano K, Kawamura H, Tanikawa T, Kawabatake H, Notani M (1982) Somatotopic arrangement of lateral spinothalamic tract in percutaneous cervical cordotomy. Appl Neurophysiol 45: 484–491
4. Onofrio BM (1970) Recent results with percutaneous cordotomy. Mayo Clin Proc 45: 689–694
5. Taira T, Amano K, Kawamura H, Tanikawa T (1985) Cerebral evoked responses elicited by direct stimulation of the lateral spinothalamic tract in the human. Appl Neurophysiol 48: 267–270
6. Taren JA, Davis R, Crosby EC (1969) Target physiologic corroboration in stereotaxic cervical cordotomy. J Neurosurg 30: 569–584
7. Tasker RR (1977) Open cordotomy. Prog Neurol Surg 8: 1–14

Correspondence: K. Amano, Department of Neurosurgery, Neurological Institute, Tokyo Women's Medical College, 8-1 Kawada-cho, Shinjuku-ku, Tokyo, Japan.

Biological Research in Psychiatry

Acta Neurochirurgica, Suppl. 52, 149–153 (1991)

The Functional Approach of Biological Research in Psychiatry

J.J. López-Ibor Jr.

Department of Psychiatry, Hospital Ramon Y Cajal, Madrid, Spain

Summary

When neurobiological investigation looks beyond nosological perspectives into the search for correlations between isolated symptoms or specific behaviour patterns (some of which may be normal) and laboratory findings, many controversies seem to become clear. A paradigm of this approach is the Serotonin (5-HT) involvement in a wide range of psychiatric disorders and specific behaviour patterns all of them characterized by a poor control of impulses. Psychopharmacotherapy with substances able to interfere with the metabolism of this neurotransmitter, mostly antidepressants, are able to compensate what appear to be very dissimilar conditions. Therefore, the hypothesis that Serotonin is important for the control of impulses is a key to the interpretation of many findings and to the penetration of the complex field of biological substrate of psycho (patho) logy.

Keywords: Serotonin; suicide; impulsivity; aggressivity.

Abbreviations: Serotonin (5-HT); 5-Hydroxy-indole-acetic acid (5-HIAA); Homovanilic acid (HVA); Noradrenaline (NA); Dopamine (DA); Tryptophan (TP); 5-Hydroxy-tryptophan (5-HTP); Tyramine (TYR); Clomipramine (CMI); Cerebro-spinal fluid (CSF); Metoxi-hydroxyphenyl-glycol (MHPG); Dexamethasone suppression test (DST); Prolactin (PRL); Methyl-chloro-phenyl-piperazine (m-CPP).

The basic problem of biological research in psychiatry is how to correlate biological findings with clinical data. In the following, the role of 5-HT in psychiatric disorder and behaviour will be reviewed as a paradigm for the rest of neurotransmitters and neuromodulators involved in psychological activity. Most of what we know about 5-HT and psychopathology has its origin in research of mood disorders, and here several perspectives have dominated the field for years. In a first approach a discussion arose on "the" neurochemical background of depressions. A serotonergic theory[24] had to face a noradrenergic one[58], with conflicting data in favour of one or the other. Later on several groups tried to identify "neurochemical families" of depressive disorders such as type A, or serotonergic, responding to imipramine and related ("5-HT") antidepressants and a type B, or noradrenergic, responding better to noradrenergic antidepressants such as nortryptilline [44,29]. Such theories never had an impact on every day practice, and the earlier research with selective reuptake blockers of 5-HT such as with zimeldine, failed to identify a "serotonergic" depression.

Although old in time, Birkmayer's hypothesis[12] is very modern. Looking at the serum concentrations of TYR, the aminoacid precursor of the cathecolamines and TP, a precursor of 5-HT (quite a crude way of looking at the problem for today's standards) he found that depressive patients had concentrations outside the normal range for TYR, TP or both, postulating that an imbalance in the tonus of both systems was responsible for the clinical picture, rather than abnormal values of one or the other. With a certain success they postulated TP treatment for the depression and other side effects such as confusion presenting themselves during 1-DOPA treatment for Parkinson's disease.

Beyond these methodological difficulties, in the last few years a new perspective has appeared which is having a high impact on research. It is characterised not by the attempt to look for the substrate, or the type or the unbalance present in specific disorders but by another more challenging approach. In CSF studies on patients with a wide range of diagnoses, Banki *et al.*[6–10] found that the presence of some symptoms coincided with specific neurochemical variations, independent of the clinical diagnosis. For instance, suicidal behaviour coincided with low concentration of 5-HIAA, the catabolite of 5-HT, delusions with high concentrations of HVA, the metabolite of NA and psychomotor inhibition with low concentrations of HVA. This approach bears a strong relationship to the concept of target symptoms[27] to describe the fact that psychotropic medication does lessen some symptoms of disorders and some do not.

5-HT has been claimed to be involved in a wide range of psychiatric conditions and also in specific behaviours which by themselves cannot be considered as pathological. Besides the affective disorders, both depressive and manic and both in the full blown episodes as well as during the intervals (supposedly as traits of vulnerability to relapses), several others should be considered. Alterations in the metabolism of 5-HT have been described in: obsessive-compulsive disorders, suicidal behaviour, aggressivity, eating disorders, alcoholism, anxiety disorders (i.e.: panic attacks) and in weather related dysthymias. (See for a revision of the literature, 42). But the list is not complete, as 5-HT is also involved in sleep[37], pain and analgesia, attention deficit disorders[36], hyperkinetic syndrome related to the so called "minimal brain dysfunction"[67], and psychotic syndromes of childhood[19] probably due to an increase in tissue tryptophan uptake and use[36], sexual behaviour, in several other conditions in which the central nervous system is involved (phenylketonuria, 52; migraine, 59; hypotonia in Down's syndrome, 56; Alzheimer's disease and convulsions) and in many in which it is not the case[51]. To make the situation even more complicated, other 5-HT metabolites or structurally related substances have been claimed to be involved in their role as false neurotransmitters in delusions and psychedelic phenomena, such as in the case of LSD[46] or of 5-hydroxytryptolines in delusions related to alcoholism[26].

It is even more interesting to observe that the specific correlations between neurochemical findings and clinical symptoms has been expanded to behaviour patterns of normal subjects, or at least of individuals who by no means do deserve a psychiatric diagnosis. We are confronted here with a unitarian perspective on psychology and psychopathology, which has been refereed to as psycho (patho) logy in German phenomenological psychiatry[13,38] and in Spanish psychiatry[22].

Such a wide range of conditions first gives rise to the question of how specific the involvement of 5-HT is, and how many artifacts are present in this approach to investigation. Nevertheless, good evidence exists that 5-HT has some specific relationships to clinical psychiatry which are worth pursuing beyond strong methodological difficulties.

Post-mortem studies show an increase in the number of 5-HT receptors in frontal cortex of suicide victims[61] and a reduced β adrenergic receptor binding, although in violent suicide victims the number of 5-HT binding sites are within normal limits[45]. Moreover, there is a reduction of presynaptic imipramine binding sites on serotonergic terminals in frontal cortex of suicide victims[53,60] and a decrease in MAO activity in alcoholic victims of suicide[30]. All these findings are suggestive of a reduced presynaptic 5-HT activity leading to a compensatory upregulation of postsynaptic binding sites in victims of suicide. It also appears to be a concomitant reduction of presynaptic noradrenergic activity.

Platelet studies essentially suggest the same hypothesis: Several authors[17,31,68] have found low platelet MAO activity in patients with suicidal behaviour and others[66] have found an increased number of binding sites in the same type of patients.

CSF research has yielded very significant results. The most significant correlations are those of suicidal attempts and low 5-HIAA concentration, and delusional symptoms and psychomotor retardation and low HVA concentration. On the other hand, Åsberg *et al.*[1,2,3,4,5] have published a series of papers in which they describe a correlation between violent suicidal behaviour and low concentrations of 5-HIAA in CSF. These same authors have suggested that this relationship has to do with aggressive behaviour in general. Basically, suicide is a form of self aggressivity in not deprived of a certain heteroaggressivity (suicides for revenge, etc.). Brown *et al.*[15,16] have published concordant evidence with the above-mentioned in affective disorders, and other researchers in schizophrenic patients[55,39,49], in personality disorders[14,15], in anxiety disorders[66] and in violent, impulsive offenders who, in comparison with offenders who have meditated and prepared their violent criminal action, have lower concentrations of 5-HIAA in CSF[40]. Even more interesting is the correlation of low concentrations of 5-HIAA in CSF and hostility scores in the Rorschach test[57] or in impulsivity and sensation-seeking behaviour[50]. These publications suggest the importance of serotonin transmission in behaviours apparently very different such as suicide, aggressivity and lack of control of impulses.

CSF has yielded data on other neurotransmitters and substances both of which point again to the involvement of other systems or to the unspecific presence of anxiety or stress: low concentrations of HVA, the catabolite of DA[8,47,48,65,68], low Mg and 5-HT[11], low melatonin[68] and high MHPG (the catabolite of the cathecolamines) in suicidal patients with anxiety, agitation, somatisation and insomnia[55].

Research on suicide and aggressivity, even the most biological one, has to take into account social factors, since the incidence of one or the other is very different in different environments. Nevertheless the findings mentioned are present in research carried out both in countries with a high (Hungary, Sweden) as well as a low (USA, Spain) incidence of suicide.

Stress by itself, as measured by modification of the controls of secretion of cortisol, has been related with suicidal behaviour. An early paper by Bunney *et al.*[18] showed a positive correlation of suicidal behaviour and a high urinary excretion of 17-OH-corticosteroids and what is more interesting, this finding had a highly predictive value (to be found only in some 5-HIAA CSF studies). Coryell and Schlesser[25] have described an abnormal DST response in suicidal behaviour, which has been reported also by others[28,68] together with a blunted TSH response to TRH[68].

Our own findings[41]throw some light on this field. In a sample of patients suffering from major depression with melancholia, in which a trial of the clinical response to 5-HTP (plus carbidopa) was undertaken, we found that those with a history of suicidal behaviour or strong suicidal ideation had lower concentrations of 5-HIAA in CSF than those in which they were absent (9.1 ng/ml vs 16.8 ng/ml). In the suicidal group the number of non-suppressors to the DST was significantly higher (in accordance with several other studies[21,25,63]), and the mean baseline cortisol concentration in peripheral blood and in CSF was also higher than in the group of patients with low scores in the suicidal items. Furthermore, the fact of being suicidal was a good predictor of a positive response to the 5-HTP treatment, therefore suggesting the presence of a 5-HT alteration which could be corrected with a 5-HT precursor in those patients. In our sample, a treatment with 5-HTP was able to significantly increase the concentration in CSF of 5-HIAA but also of HVA. It is impossible to conclude whether the HVA increases (which had also previously been described earlier[65] is due to the direct effect of the 5-HTP or to an indirect one (i.e., increase in physical activity or other). Montgomery *et al.*[47,48] have described in impulsive suicidal behaviour, a superior action of flupentixol, a neuroleptic, than the one with mianserine, which suggests that dopamine may also be involved in suicide. Carlson *et al.*[20] postulate that the NA system is involved in drive and retardation and 5-HT system in dysphoric mood. Pfeiffer[54] postulates that depression is related to a decreased 5-HT and an increased histamine metabolism and impulsivity to a decreased 5-HT metabolism, a decreased degradation of cathecholamines, and in both cases, stress is a significant factor (the latter can be related to DST and cortisol concentration in blood and CSF findings).

In personality disorders with physical aggression and motor impulsivity, a blunted PRL response to the fenfluramine challenge has been found[23]; again, this relates to a possible 5-HT deficit. We have published the same finding together with a particular pattern in the cortisol response to fenfluramine in comparison with age and sex matched controls. Borderline suicidal patients show high cortisol baseline concentrations (suggesting a high level of stress) and a very blunted response to the challenge (suggesting a reduced ability to respond to external stresses)[43]. Others[62] have described a reduction of 3H-imipramine binding sites on platelets of children with conduct disorders suggesting again the importance of a disturbed presynaptic serotonergic activity in heterogenous populations of non-depressed psychiatric patients characterized by a reduction of behaviourial constraints.

In any case all this data strongly suggest that : a) A decrease in 5-HT metabolism is related not only to depression in general but also to some specific symptoms of depression and of other disorders, mainly suicidal behaviour and impulsivity. The positive response of treatments that enhance 5-HT metabolism (i.e., zimeldine,[47,48]) is concordant with this hypothesis, b) Specific neurotransmitter systems do not function in isolation and more often than not, several alterations are found in clinical syndromes, and c) Stress, as measured by DST or cortisol concentrations in body fluids, plays an unspecific and almost always present role.

It is interesting that Insel *et al.*[32,33,34,35] have described in obsessive patients a transitory increase in their symptomatology immediately after the administration of m-CPP, although an obsessive disorder is a condition where serotonergic antidepressants have proven to have a therapeutical effect. This observation can be interpreted as the result of a hypersensitivity of the postsynaptic receptors, compensatory of a functional presynaptic deficit.

Beyond the methodological difficulties mentioned, the wide range of conditions in which 5-HT is claimed to be involved, different methods give coinciding evidence and a certain common trait evolves from a high background noise. The studies in suicide and aggressivity point towards a decrease inserotonergic functions in those cases where the behaviour involved is violent or not premeditated, and, therefore, the 5-HT involvement in the control of impulses in such patients has been suggested [47,48]. This hypothesis could explain the findings in bulimia, alcoholism and perhaps self-destructive behaviour.

Furthermore, a basic principle of the target symptoms or patterns approach is that the same neurotransmitter may be involved in many psycho (patho) logical features and that many of these patterns are related to the same neurotransmitter. Again, we have to forget about "specificity", even more causal specificity, to consider the complex interactions of a multifactorial homeostatic equilibrium controlled by integrative systems of a high complexity.

References

1. Åsberg M, Träskman L, Thoren, P (1976a) 5-HIAA in the cerebro-spinal fluid – a biochemical suicide predictor? Arch Gen Psychiatry 33: 1193–1197
2. Åsberg M, Thoren P, Träskman-Bendz, L (1976b) Serotonin depression: a biochemical subgroup within the affective disorders? Science 191: 478–480
3. Åsberg M, Bertilsson L (1979) Serotonin in depressive illness – studies of CSF 5-HIAA. In: B Saletu (ed) Neuropsychopharmacology Pergamon Press, Oxford 105–115.
4. Åsberg M, Edman G, Rydin, E, Schalling D, Träskman-Bendz L, Wagner A (1984a) Biological correlates of suicidal behaviour. Clin Neuropharmacol 7 [Suppl] 1: 758–759
5. Åsberg M, Bertilsson L, Martensson B, Scalia-Tomba GP, Thoren P, Träskman-Bendz L (1984b) CSF monoamine metabolites in melancholia. Acta Psychiatrica Scandinavica 69: 201–219
6. Banki CM, Arato M (1983) Amine metabolites and neuroendrocrine responses related to depression and suicide. J Affective Disord 5: 223–232
7. Banki CM (1977) Correlation between cerebrospinal fluid amine metabolites and psychosomatic activity in affective disorders. J Neurochem 28: 255–257
8. Banki CM, Molnar G (1981a) Cerebrospinal fluid 5-hydroxyindoleacetic acid as an index of central serotonergic processes. Psychiatr Res 5: 23–32
9. Banki CM, Molnar, G, Vojnik M (1981b) Cerebrospinal fluid amine metabolites, tryptophan and clinical parameters in depression. Part 2: Psychopathological symptoms. J Affective Disord 3: 91–99
10. Banki CM, Molnar G, Fekete I (1981c) Correlation of individual symptoms and other clinical variables with cerebrospinal fluid amine metabolites and tryptophan in depression. Archiv für Psychiatrie und Nervenkrankheiten 229: 343–353
11. Banki CM, Arato M, Papp Z, Kurcz M (1984) Biochemical markers in suicidal patients. J Affective Disord 6: 341–350
12. Birkmayer W, Linauer W (1970) Störungen des Tyrosin und Tryptophan-Metabolismus bei Depressionen. Archiv für Psychiatrie und Nervenkrankheiten 213: 377–387
13. Blankenburg W (1969) Ansätze zu einer Psychopathologie des "common sense". Confinia Psychiatrica 12: 144–163
14. Brown GL, Goodwin FK, Ballenger JC *et al* (1978) Aggression in humans correlates with cerebrospinal fluid amine metabolites. Psychiatry Res 1: 131–139
15. Brown GL, Ebert MH, Goyer PF, Jimerson DC, Klein WJ, Bunney WE, Goodwin FK (1982) Aggression, suicide and serotonin: relationship to CSF amine metabolites. Am J Psychiatry 139: 741–746
16. Brown GL, Goodwin FK (1984) Diagnostic, clinical and personality characteristics of aggressive men with low 5-HIAA. Clin Neuropharm 7 [Suppl] 1: 407–408
17. Buschsbaum MS, Coursey RD, Murphy DL (1976) The biochemical high-risk paradigm-behavioural and familial correlates of low platelet monoamine oxidase activity. Science 194: 339–341
18. Bunney WE, Fawcett JA (1965) Possibility of a biochemical test for suicidal potential. Arch Gen Psychiatry 13: 232–239
19. Campbell M, Friedman E, De Vine (1974) Blood serotonin in psychotic and brain damaged children. J Autism and Childhood Schizophrenia 4: 33–41
20. Carlsson A, Corrodi H, Fuxe K, Hokfelt T (1969) Effects of some antidepressant drugs on the depletion of intraneuronal brain catecholamine stores caused by 4,α-dimethyl-meta-tyramine. Eur J Pharmacol 5: 367–3730
21. Carroll BJ, Greden JF, Feinberg M (1981) Suicide, neuroendocrine dysfunction and CSF 5-HIAA concentrations in depression. In: Angrist, Burrows, Lader, Lingjaerde, Sedvall, Wheatley (eds) Recent Advances in Neuropsychopharmacology. Pergamon Press, Oxford pp 181–197
22. Castilla Del Pino C (1978) Introducción a la Psiquiatría. 1. Problemas generales de Psico (pato) logia. Madrid: Alianza.
23. Coccaro EM, Siever LJ, Klar M, Rubinstein R, Moskovitz A, Davis KL (1986) 5-HT in affective and personality disorders. In Abstracts of the ACNP Congress. San Juan, PR, December
24. Coppen A, Shaw DM, Farrell JP (1963) Potentiation of the antidepressive effect of a monoamino-oxidose inhibitor by tryptophan. Lancet 1: 79–87
25. Coryell W, Schlesser MA (1981) Suicide and the dexamethasone suppression test in unipolar depression. Am J Psychiatry 138: 1120–1121
26. Davis VE, Brown H, Huff JA, Cashaw JL (1967) The alteration of serotonin metabolism to 5-hydroxytryptophol by ethanol ingestion in man. J Lab Clin Med 69: 132
27. Freyhan FA (1979) The target symptoms for treatment of depressive illness revisited. Compr Psychiatry 20: 495–501
28. Fusté R, Martinez Pina A, Monne J (1986) Expresión psicoendocrina de la conducta suicida. Estudio psiocoendocrinológico en dos grupos de pacientes suicidas. Actas Luso-Españolas de Neurologia, Psiquiatría Y Ciencias Afines 14: 369–378
29. Goodwin FK, Cowdry RW, Webster MH (1978) Predictors of drug response in the affective disorders: toward an integrated approach. In: Lipton MA, DiMascio A, Killam KE (eds) Psychopharmacology: A question of progress. Raven Press, New York, pp 1277–1288
30. Gottfries G, Oreland L, Wiberg A, Winblad B (1975) Lowered monoamine oxidase activity in brain from alcoholic suicides. J Neurochem 25: 667–673
31. Gottfries G, Von Knorring L, Oreland L (1980) Platelet monoamine oxidase activity in patients with suicidal behaviour and in subgroups of affective psychosis. Prog Neuropsychopharmacol 185: 192
32. Insel TR, Roy BF, Cohen RM (1982) Possible development of the serotonin syndrome in man. Am J Psychiatry 139: 954–955
33. Insel T (1982) Antiobsessional and antidepressant effects of clomipramine in the treatment of obsessive-compulsive disorder. Psychopharmacol Bull 18 (4): 115–117

34. Insel T (1983) Obsessive-compulsive disorder. A double-blind trail of clomipramine and clorgyline. Arch Gen Psychiatry 40: 605–612
35. Insel T, Mueller EA, Alterman I (1985) Obsessive-compulsive disorder and serotonin: Is there a connection? Biol Psychiatry 20: 1174–1188
36. Irwin M, Belendink K, Mccloskey K, Freedman DF (1981) Tryptophan metabolism in children with attentional deficit disorders. Am J Psychiatry 138: 1082–1085
37. Jouvet M (1969) Biogenic amines and the states of sleep. Science 163: 32–41
38. Kisker KP (1969) Phenomenologie der Intersubtektivität, Handbuch der Psychologie. In: Gronmann (ed) Sozialpsychologie Vol 7/1. Hofgrefe, Gottingen pp 321–362
39. Levy AB, Kurtz N, Kling AS (1984) Association between cerebral ventricular enlargement and suicide attempts in chronic schizophrenia. Am J Psychiatry 141: 438–439
40. Linnoila M, Virkkunen M, Scheinin M, Muutila A, Rimon R, Goodwin FK (1984) Low cerebrospinal fluid 5-hydroxyindoleacetic acid concentration differentiates impulsive from non-impulsive violent behaviour. Life Sciences 33: 2609–2414
41. Lopez-Ibor Jr JJ, Saiz-Ruiz J, Perez de los Cobos JC (1985) Biological correlations of suicide and aggressivity in major depressions (with melancholia): 5-hidroxyindoleacetic acid and cortisol in cerebral spinal fluid, dexamethasone suppression test and therapeutic response to 5-hydroxytryptophan. Neuropsychobiology 67–74
42. Lopez-Ibor Jr JJ (1988) The involvement of serotonin in psychiatric disorders and behavior. Br J Psychiatry 153 [Suppl]: 26–39
43. Lopez-Ibor Jr JJ, Lana F, Saiz J (1990) Serotonin, impulsivity and suicidal behavior. In: Proceedings of the VIII World Congress of Psychiatry. Athens (in press)
44. Maas JW, Fawcett JA, Dekirmenjian H (1972) Catecholamine metabolism depressive illness and drug response. Arch Gen Psychiatry 26: 252–262
45. Mann JJ, Stanley M, Mcbride P A, Mcewen B S (1986) Increased serotonin$_2$ and β-adrenergic receptor binding in the prontal corticols of suicide victims. Arch Gen Psychiatry 43: 954–959
46. Mantegazzinni P (1960) Pharmacological actions of indolealkylamins and precursor amino acids on the central nervous system. Handbuch der experimentelle Pharmacologie 19: 424, Springer, Berlin
47. Montgomery SA, Montgomery D (1982a) Pharmacological prevention of suicidal behaviour. J Affective Disord 4: 291–298
48. Montgomery SA, Montgomery DB (1982b) Drug treatment of suicidal behaviour. In: Costa E, Racagnli G, (eds) Typical and a typical antidepressants: clinical practice. Raven Press, New York, pp 349–355
49. Ninan PT, Van Kamen DP, Cheinin M, Linnoila M, Bunney WE, Goodwin FK (1984) CSF 5-hydroxyindole acetic acid levels in suicidal schizophrenic patients. Am J Psychiatry 141: 566–569
50. Oreland L, Wiberg A, Åsberg M, Traskman L, Sjostrand L, Thoren P, Bertilsson L, Tybring G (1981) Platelet MAO activity and monoamine metabolism in CSF in depressed and suicidal patients and in healthy controls. Psychiatry Res 4: 21–29
51. Page IH (1968) Serotonin. Yearbook Medical Publishers, Chicago
52. Pare CMB, Sandler M, Staley RS (1957) 5-hydroxy-tryptamine deficiency in phenyliketonuria. Lancet i: 1099
53. Perry GK, Marshall EF, Blessed G, Tomlinson BE, Perry RH (1983) Decrease imipramine binding in the brains of patients with depressive illness. Br J Psychiatry 142: 188–192
54. Pfeiffer CC, Bacchi D (1975) Copper, zinc, manganese, niacin, and pyridoxine in the schizophrenias. J Appl Nutrition 27: 9–39
55. Remond Jr DE, Katz MM, Maas JW, Casper R, Davis JM (1986) Cerebrospinal fluid amine metabolites. Relationships with behavioural measurements in depressed, manic, and healthy control subjects. Arch Gen Psychiatry 43: 939–947
56. Rosner F, Ong BH, Paine RS, Mahanand D (1965) Blood-serotonin activity in trisomic and translocation Down's syndrome. Lancet i: 1191
57. Rydin E, Schalling D, Åsberg M (1982) Rorschach ratings in depressed and suicidal patients with low CSF 5-HIAA. Psychiatry Res 1: 229–243
58. Schildkraut JJ (1965) The catecholamine hypothesis of affective disorders: a review of supporting evidence. Am J Psychiatry 122: 509–522
59. Sicuteri F (1959) Prophylactic and therapeutic properties of 1-methyl-lysergic acid etanolamide in migrane. Arch Allergy 15: 300
60. Stanley M, Gershon VJ (1982) Tritiated imipramine binding sites are decreased in the frontal cortex of suicides. Science 216: 1337–1339
61. Stanley M, Mann JJ (1983) Serotonin-^{2} binding sites are increased in the frontal cortex of suicide victims. Lancet i: 214–216
62. Stoff DM, Pollock L, Vitiello B, Berhar D, Bridger WH (1987) Reduction of (^{3}H)-imipramine binding sites on platelets of conduct-disordered children. Neuropsychopharmacology 1: 55–62
63. Targum SD, Rosen L, Capodanno AE (1983) The dexamethasone suppression test in suicidal patients with unipolar depression. Am J Psychiatry 140: 877–879
64. Träskman L, Tybring G, Åsberg M, Bertilsson L, Lanto O, Schalling D (1980) Cortisol in the CSF of depressed and suicidal patients. Arch Gen Psychiatry 37: 761–766
65. van Praag HM (1983) CSF 5-HIAA and suicide in non depressed schizophrenics. Lancet ii: 977–978
66. Wägner A, Aberg-Wistedt A, Åsberg M, Ekquist B, Martensson B, Montero D (1985) Low (^{3}H)-imipramine binding in platelets from untreated depressed patients compared to healthy controls. Psychiatry Res 16: 131–139
67. Wender PH (1969) Platelet serotonin levels in children with "minimal brain dysfunction". Lancet ii: 1021
68. Ziporyn T (1983) Depression, violent suicide tied to low metabolite level. J Am Med Assoc 250: 3141–3142

Correspondence: J.J. López-Ibor, Jr., Department of Psychiatry, Hospital Ramon y Cajal Carretera de Colmeuar. E-28034 Madrid, Spain.

Epilepsy

Acta Neurochirurgica, Suppl. 52, 157–160 (1991)

Surgical Treatment for Epilepsy. Results After a Minimum Follow-up of Five Years

R. Garcia Sola[2] and **J. Miravet**[1]

Department of Clinical Neurophysiology, Hospital Puerta de Hierro, and [2]Department of Neurosurgery, Hospital de la Princessa, Autonomous University, Madrid, Spain

Summary

Forty-two patients have been surgically treated for medically uncontrollable epilepsy, using the Talairach and Bancaud methodology. The mean age of the patients was 19 years (range 6–54 years). The location of the epileptogenic zone was: frontal in 18 patients, temporal in 14, temporo-parieto-occipital junction in 4, parietal in 4 and occipital in 2.

The overall surgical results are: 20 patients are seizure free and 6 patients had occasional seizures (62% success rate). There has been a significant decrease in the number of seizures in 12 patients. The seizures persist in 4 patients.

Only two patients, both with a parietal focus, presented additional postoperative neurological deficit (mild paresis in the contralateral lover limb). This was preoperatively foreseen, and accepted by the patient, on guarantees of the removal of the epileptogenic zone and amelioration of seizures.

Keywords: Epilepsy; medically uncontrollable epilepsy; surgical treatment of epilepsy; stereoelectroencephalography.

Introduction

Surgical treatment of epilepsy continues to be a subject of controversy. There are numerous ways to approach the problem, and the most commonly used techniques are the following:

1. *Stereotactic Lesion Techniques* – Introduced by E. A. Spiegel and H.T. Wycis[6] they can be subdivided into:

a) Lesions located in subcortical nuclei, intended to reduce the cortical excitability;
b) Destruction of a region presumed to be responsible for the triggering of the epileptic discharge; and
c) Section of the principal propagation pathways of the discharge. (e.g. section of the corpus callosum).[9]

2. *Stimulation Techniques* – Introduced by Cooper[1], currently of more theoretical than practical importance.

3. *Cortical Resection* – The cortical area to be resected is identified using two different neurophysiological methods: the methodology developed by Penfield and Jasper in 1954[5], based on electrocorticography, and the Talairach and Bancaud[8] methodology based on stereoelectroencephalography. The latter one aims at a better definition of the epileptic focus, by the study of its functional temporo-spatial profile in a three-dimensional anatomical conception.

Our team elaborated a program for the surgical treatment of epileptic patients in whom medical treatment was unsuccessful, following the Talairach and Bancaud[8] methodology. The purpose of this communication is to report the long-term results.

Material and Methods

The main phases of the surgical treatment of the epileptic patient were the following:

A. Patient Selection – The basic concepts did not vary from those set forth by other authors and which can be summarized as follows:

1. Pharmaceutically uncontrollable epilepsy;
2. Seizures interfere seriously with the patient's life style;
3. The patient is sufficiently motivated and collaborative;
4. The functional study confirms the existence of partial epilepsy; and
5. It is likely that the resection of the epileptogenic zone (EZ) will not produce serious, incapacitating neurological deficits.

B. Electroclinical Study (ECS) – An EEG and clinical analysis of the interictal period as well as the semiology of spontaneous seizures were performed. These were recorded by synchronized video-tape and EEG system. With the obtained data, a hypothesis was formulated with respect to the anatomo-functional location of the origin of the seizures, as well as their probable propagation pathways.

C. Stereoencephalographic Study (SEG) – Stereotactic bilateral carotid angiography and ventriculography were performed[7]. A cerebral map is drawn for each patient, based on the AC–PC intercommissural line. To this diagram we added the data obtained from the CT scan. This has been of great use to define the limits of a porencephalic cavity, to locate a lesion undetectable by other means, or to obtain a three-dimensional view of a large and convoluted lesion (Figs. 1, 2).

D. Stereoelectroencephalographic Study (SEEG) – Depth. electrodes were placed in accordance with the location of the epileptic focus and with the help of anatomical data obtained by the previous studies. This allowed us to perform a three-dimensional EEG of the seizures, whether spontaneous or provoked by stimulation. The global purpose of the SEEG is to delineate the epileptogenic zone (EZ), the lesion (LZ), the irritative zone (IZ), the propagation pathways and the function of the explored areas as accurately as possible.

E. Cortical Resection – A resection was performed of the EZ and LZ previously delineated by SEEG, preserving important vessels visualised with the aid of angiography (Figs. 1,2).

F. Postoperative Follow-up – In most of the patients a clinical examination, EEG and CT scan, as well as the plasma levels of antiepileptic drugs have been performed every 6 months for the first 2 years and every year thereafter. The medication was not modified until one and a half postoperative year had elapsed.

G. Assessment of Results – The first 42 operated patients have been classified in 4 groups[8]:

1. Seizure-free (S.F.).
2. Occasional Seizures (E.S.), upon discontinuing medication and/or after alcohol ingestion.
3. Significant decrease (S.D.) of the number of seizures, to at least one tenth of the number of preoperative seizures, with a clear improvement in their daily life.
4. The persistence (P) of seizures prevents the patients from having any improvement in the quality of life.

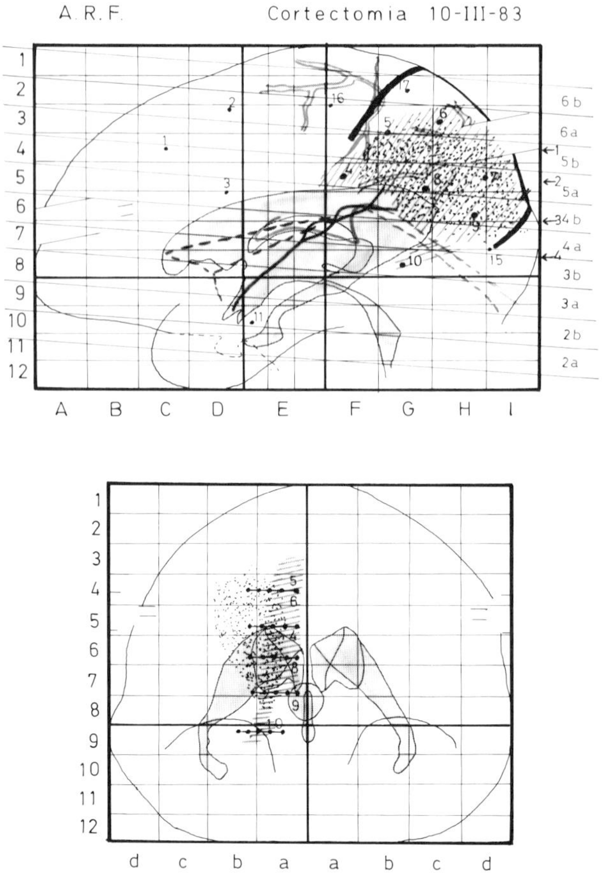

Fig. 1. A.R.F. 24-year-old patient with post-traumatic epilepsy. Cerebral lesion observed in the CT scan (dotted area)

Results

The mean age of the patients was 18.7 years (range 6–54). The clinical records and pathological analyses confirmed the etiology in 69% of the cases: birth trauma or anoxia (6 pts.), head injury (6 pts.), post-inflammatory scarring (5 pts.), tumour (7 pts.) and vascular malformations (5 pts.).

The global results at the end of a minimum postoperative follow-up of 5 years and a maximum of 12.1/2 years have been: 20 patients are seizure-free; 6 patients have had exceptional seizures (1–3 seizures in all the postoperative period). This means a global surgical success among 62% of the patients. There was a significant decrease of seizures in 12 patients and no improvement in the rest (Table 1).

In relation to the location of the E.Z. the percentage of surgical success (S. F. or E.S.) was: 18 patients with frontal E.Z., from which 9 (50%) are seizure-free; 14 temporal epilepsies, 11 (78.5%) without seizures; 4 parietal epilepsies, all seizure-free; (100%); 4 patients with E.Z. at the temporoparieto-occipital junction (T.P.O.), from which only 1 is seizure free; and, finally 2 patients with occipital E.Z. and one seizure-free.

In relation to the results obtained after the SEEG study, the patients can be classified into three groups:

A. – Patients with a correct delineation of the E.Z.: surgical success in 22 out of 26 patients (85%).

B. – Patients with an insufficient E.Z. definition. surgical success in 3 out of 9 patients (33%).

C. – Patients with bilateral E.Z. (5 frontal and 2 temporal): only 1 patient with temporal epilepsy is seizure-free.

Excluding the last group of bilateral E.Z., the relationship between demonstrable lesions in the CT scan and the surgical results have been studied in 35 patients with a single E.Z. In 23 patients with no lesion (16 pts.) or small (2 < cm) (7 pts.), complete remission of epilepsy was achieved in all except 1 patient with

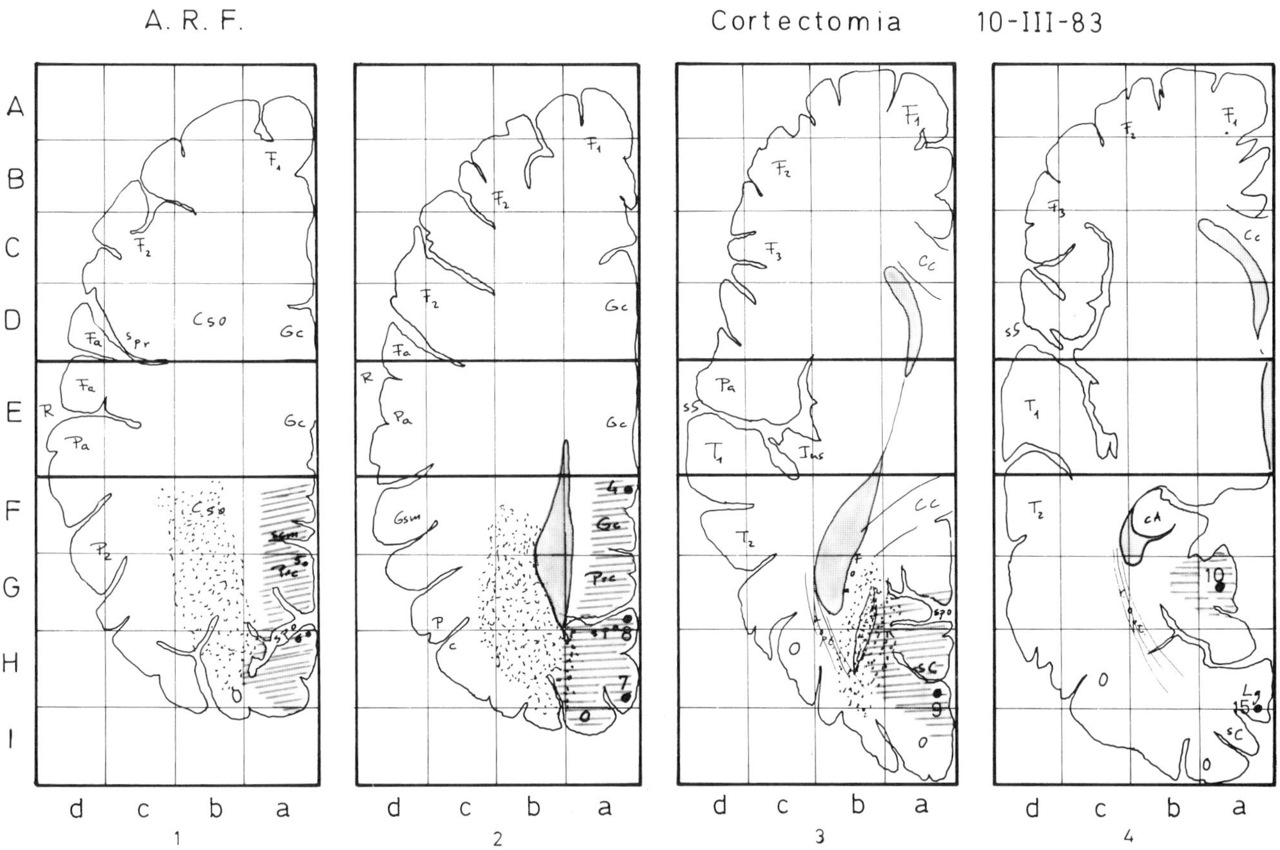

Fig. 2. Same patient as in Fig. 1. Axial views at different levels (1–4). The internal parieto-occipital cortex to be resected can be seen (shaded area)

Table 1. *Surgical results. Seizure-free (S.F.), Exceptional Seizures (E.S.), Significant Decrease (S.D.), Persistence (P). See text*

LOCATION	N	S.F.	E.S.	S.D.	P
FRONTAL	18	6 [5] (6)	3 [3] (3)	6 [1] (2) ⟨2⟩	3 ⟨3⟩
TEMPORAL	14	9 [8] (7) ⟨1⟩	2 [2] (2)	3 (2) ⟨1⟩	0
PARIETAL	4	3 [2] (2)	1	0	0
T.P.O.	4	1 [1] (1)	0	2	1
OCCIPITAL	2	1 [1] (1)	0	1	0
TOTAL PATIENTS	42 [23] (26) ⟨7⟩	20 [17] (17) ⟨1⟩	6 [5] (5)	12 [1] (4) ⟨3⟩	4 ⟨3⟩

[] Number of patients with no lesion or small lesion
() Number of patients with correct definition of Epileptogenic zone
⟨⟩ Number of patients with bilateral Epileptogenic zone

frontal epilepsy who remains with significant decrease of seizures.

Discussion

The mean age at operation, etiology and the global surgical results are similar to those of Talairach and Bancaud[8]. The results are influenced by many factors which cannot be completely defined because of the small number of patients. However, we would like to stress some points that are of importance:

A. – With regard to the E.Z. location, temporal and parietal epilepsies were the most successful. This is probably due to the obvious clinical features in this form of epilepsy and the fact that a relatively small cortical field has to be explored.

B. – When the E.Z. is not well delimited, due to errors, technical short-comings of the preoperative exploration or to the wide extension of the E.Z., the percentage of surgical success, is only 30%.

C. – Patients with bilateral epileptogenic foci have the least favourable surgical results.

D. – On analyzing the patients in relation to the lesion evident on CT scans[4], we have found that the best cases were those with no lesion of small lesion (95% of surgical successes). This could be due to three factors: the EZ was small, it was correctly delineated (in 21 out of 24 patients); and its resection was possible. As an example of the surgical limitations, two patients with parietal E.Z. had a postoperative minimal paresis of the contralateral lower extremity. This was foreseen preoperatively, and accepted by the patient, as a possible sequence to resection of the E.Z. to eradicate the seizures.

E. – The opposite may happen in cases with extensive lesions in the CT scan. Then, unsatisfactory results were obtained (25% successes) because of the difficulties to correctly define the E.Z. (only 5 out of 12 patients). It was not possible to perform a complete resection of the E.Z. and L.Z. because of adjacent, critical cerebral regions.

In such cases we consider a failure when the seizures persist and there has not been at least a significant decrease. We attained our preoperative purpose in 15 patients (5 are seizures-free and 10 with significant decrease of seizures) out of 19 patients to whom we offered this palliative option.

Acknowledgements

The authors wish to express their thanks to the Funcacion Areces and to M. Messman for her translation and editorial assistance.

References

1. Cooper IS (1973) Chronic stimulation of paleocerebellar cortex in man. Lancet 1: 206
2. Garcia Sola R, Miravet J, Brasa J *et al* (1980) Relationship between the location and delimitation of the epileptic zone and surgical results. Acta Neurochir (Wien) [Suppl] 30: 117–120
3. Garcia Sola R, Miravet J, Parera C, Bravo G (1982) Curative or palliative possibilities in the surgical treatment of epileptic patients. Appl Neurophysiol 45: 471–477
4. Garcia Sola R, Miravet J, Parera C, Bravo G (1983) La TAC como factor importante de preseleccion quirurgica de pacientes con epilepsia focal grave. In: Centenario de la Neurologia en Espana. Servicio Neurologia. Hospital Santa Creu i San Pau (ed) Barcelona, Spain, pp 445–454
5. Penfield W, Jasper H (1954) Epilepsy and the functional anatomy of the human brain. Little Brown & Co, Boston
6. Spiegel EA, Wycis HT (1952) Stereoencephalotomy. Part II: Clinical and physiological applications. Grune Stratton, New York
7. Talairach J, Szikla G *et al* (1967) Atlas of stereotaxic anatomy of the telencephalon, Masson, Paris.
8. Talairach J, Bancaud J *et al* (1974) Approche nouvelle de la neurochirurgie de l' epilepsie. Neurochir (Wien) 20 [Suppl] 1
9. Van Wanegen WP, Herren RY (1940), Surgical division of commissural pathways in the corpus callosum. Relation to spread of an epileptic attack. Arch Neurol Psychiatry 44: 740–759

Correspondence: R. Garcia-Sola, Department of Neurosurgery, Hospital de la Princessa, Autonomous University, Madrid, Spain

Rezio R. Renella

Microsurgery of the Temporo-Medial Region

1989. 50 partly coloured figures.
XII, 203 pages.
Cloth DM 158,–, öS 1110,–
ISBN 3-211-82144-9

Prices are subject to change without notice

The differentiation of the temporal lobe into a lateral neocortical and a medial allocortical region is supported by developmental, anatomical and clinical evidence. Although this view of a dual temporal lobe is generally accepted by neurosurgeons dealing with functional surgery, it still receives little attention by those approaching structural abnormalities located or extending into the medio-basal region. Consequently, the characterization of the temporo-medial area as a distinct surgical region is still lacking. The major object of this study is to analyse the medial part of the temporal lobe as a distinct surgical region and to integrate the microsurgical and physiological aspects into a concept applicable to the several types of temporo-medial lesion. The study includes five sections. The first section is devoted to the morphological aspects. The second and the third sections present a simplified clinical approach to temporo-medial lesions and analyse the ancillary investigations which are indispensable for characterizing their structural and functional features. The fourth section deals with the surgical aspects of temporo-medial lesions, and especially with the selection of the optimal approach having regard to the location of a given process, and to the extent of the functional changes. The last section is devoted to commentaries concerning the neuropathological aspects and the outcome of surgery in the temporo-medial region.

Contents:

Springer-Verlag Wien New York